JUSTINE HARPER

WOMEN'S EXERCISE PROGRAMS

Unlock Your Strength and Vitality
(2024 Guide for Beginners)

Copyright © 2023 by Justine Harper

All rights reserved. No part of this publication may be reproduced, stored or transmitted in any form or by any means, electronic, mechanical, photocopying, recording, scanning, or otherwise without written permission from the publisher. It is illegal to copy this book, post it to a website, or distribute it by any other means without permission.

First edition

This book was professionally typeset on Reedsy. Find out more at reedsy.com

Contents

1	An Introduction to Female Bodybuilding	1
2	Home Exercises for Strength Training	4
3	What to Eat for Nutrition in Bodybuilding	22
4	Recipes for Healthful Eating	26
5	Advice for Novices on Strength Training	44
6	Yoga for Novices	48
7	Yoga Training Program for Novices	55
8	Yoga Training Plan for Beginners	64
9	Advice for Novices in Yoga	72

1

An Introduction to Female Bodybuilding

The Advantages of Female Strength Training

Most people believe that strength training is primarily a male activity. Because bodybuilding was associated with being "overly masculine," women frequently disapproved of the idea. Rather than this, a lot of women prefer to dedicate a significant amount of time to various forms of exercise, like cardiovascular and mild toning activities. You can't really alter the contour of your body until you begin strength training, even while these workouts can help you lose body fat and tone your muscles to some extent.

Using Strength Training to Lose Weight

All women aspire to be "hourglass shaped" and to reduce their body fat. Exercise cardio and learn how to strengthen your core muscles if you want to have this amazing body. Strength training will increase the amount of muscle in your back and shoulders, giving your upper body more definition. In addition to drawing attention to your legs and hips, strength training offers your lower body that extra flare that gives you a more voluptuous appearance. Training your biceps and triceps can assist address the issue of flabby arms, which is a complaint often voiced by women.

A strength training program for beginners will still burn fat and calories. To gain muscle, your body must perform a variety of resistance training exercises when lifting weights. Exercise like this raises your metabolism in addition to burning fat and replacing it with muscle. Your body starts to burn calories while you are at rest and during the day and night when your resting metabolism improves. In terms of weight loss, this is really beneficial. Gaining muscle requires you to burn more calories and chip away at the fat deposits that prior exercise regimens have left you with. Leaner and stronger is what strength training will make you.

Strength Training for Well-Being

Strength training has several advantages for women, one of which is that it lowers the risk of osteoporosis. Lifting weights improves your bones in addition to your muscles. By increasing bone density, it lowers the chance of bone breaks and fractures. According to research, lifting weights can strengthen and improve the health of your spine by increasing the density of the spinal bones.

Additionally, strength training helps to minimize back pain and improve posture. By strengthening your shoulders, back, and core, weight training can help you improve your posture and develop a taller, more proportionate body with straight shoulders, back, and spine. Lower back pain can also be avoided with this.

You feel happier and less stressed after doing strength exercise. Endorphins are released during weight training and activity. These neurotransmitters, called endorphins, fight depression, stop pain, and lift your spirits all around. Because endorphins excite the mind, they also increase energy and enhance attentiveness.

Strengthening Exercises

Strength training can improve your endurance, help you avoid injuries, and make other daily chores like lifting or moving objects much easier for you. Maybe you've been hesitant to start strength training because you don't want to appear Incredible Hulk-esque. Be at ease. Because hormones differ in their effects based on gender, men are more likely than women to have all that bulk. Even if you lift weights every day and increase the amount you use, as a woman you will never get the massive biceps that you see on bodybuilders. Rather, you'll appear toned, elegant, and fiercely feminine. To build a powerful, well-rounded body, pay attention to every muscle in your body.

If you haven't been motivated to start lifting weights, you should give strength training some serious thought because it has so many amazing benefits for women. It won't take long to start seeing and feeling better if you give the at-home strength training exercises in this book a try.

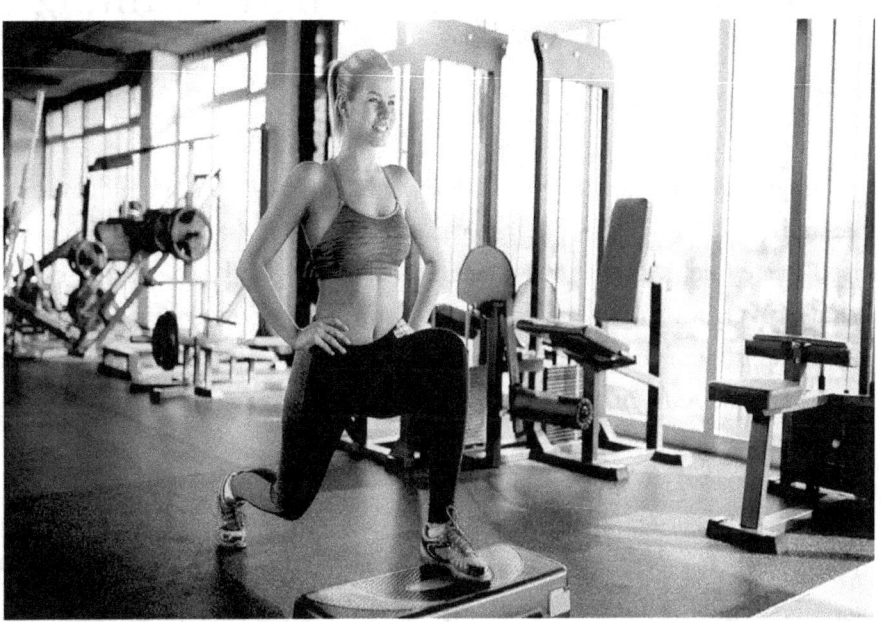

2

Home Exercises for Strength Training

Although coming to the gym is enjoyable for many bodybuilders, as a beginning, you might feel better at ease working out at home. You don't need pricey equipment or a specially designed gym to perform several fantastic weightlifting exercises in the comfort of your own home. To gain an understanding of the movements and weights you will need to lift in order to strengthen yourself, do these strength training exercises at home.

Exercises to Warm Up

It's crucial to warm up before starting a strength training program since it tells your body and mind that you're going to be engaging in some physical activity. These are a few key strategies to prepare your body for higher intensity training.

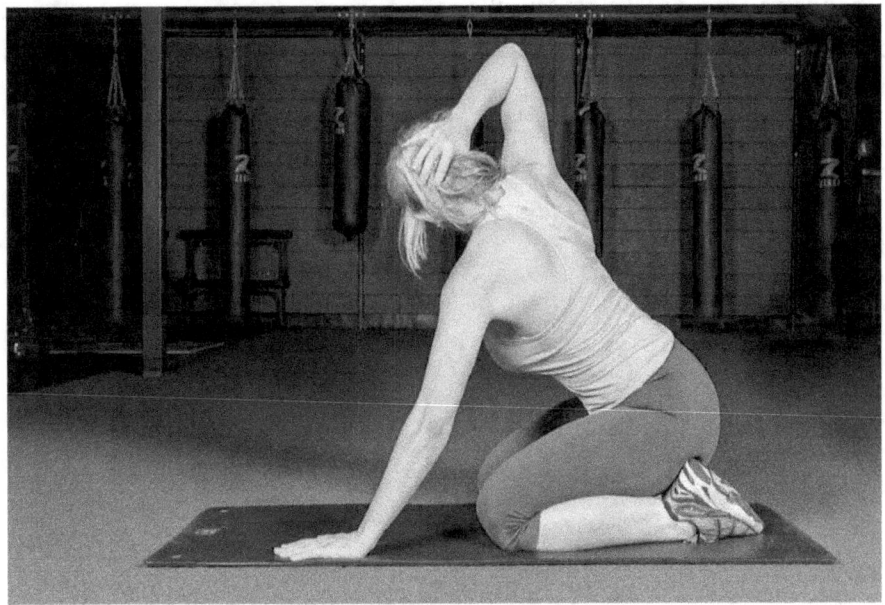

Heart rate

Warm up your body aerobically for 15 to 20 minutes at first. This will cause your heart rate to increase, your metabolism to speed up, and your muscles to become loose and heated. There are a few options available for your warm-up's cardio section; pick the one that appeals to you the most. It works best to take a quick ten-minute stroll, but if you want to step up the pace, you can even jog or even sprint. Ride a bike, perform jumping jacks, Zumba, or aerobic exercises. In order to go into the core of your weight training program, the objective is to get your body moving and raise your heart rate.

Exertion in Motion

It will help to be a little flexible. You'll discover that you can move more effectively and that your body feels more flexible as you continue to tone and shape it. You may improve your flexibility and get closer to your strength goals by stretching before and after your workouts.

1. Begin by doing some simple toe touches. Stretch your arms above your head and slowly bend at the waist while standing with your feet together. Even

though your legs will start to pull in the opposite direction, keep lowering yourself to the ground. Try putting the tips of your fingers on your toes. It's okay if you are unable to proceed that far on your first attempt. The more you put effort into it, the closer you'll get. Lift yourself back up to a standing position after a little while. Perform this five times.

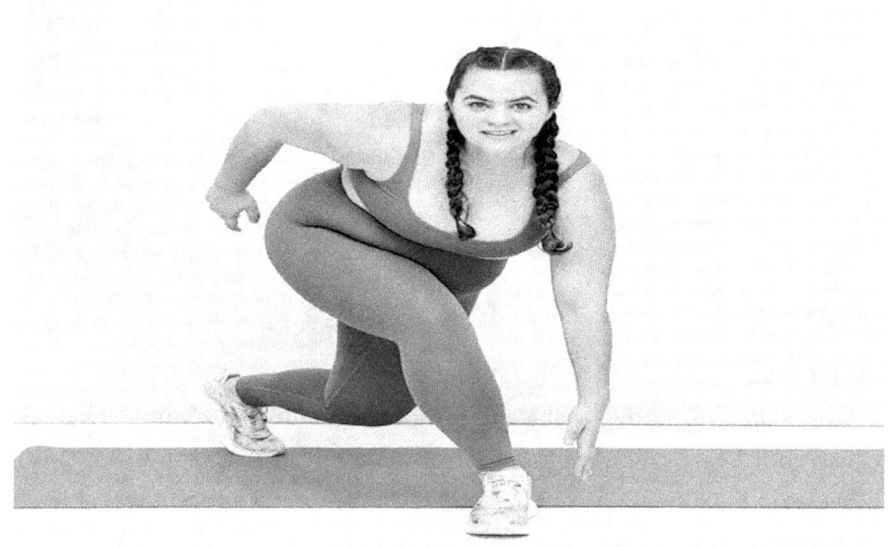

2. Proceed to perform Linear Marches and Skips. The march is a basic exercise that involves bringing your knee up to your waist and then lowering your foot to the ground. Continue with the opposite foot. Make three back-and-forth marches across the room. Next, transition it into a skip, where you hop while kicking up your knee and moving forward. While you skip three times around the room, make sure to lift your knees to your waist.

3. Next, the upper body has to warm up. Make some Arm Circles while standing with your feet shoulder-width apart. With your hands by your sides at first, raise both arms and swing them in a full circle. Perform ten swings in each direction: ten forward swings and ten backward swings.

Equilibrium

Learning how to balance your body weight and maintain focus should be a part of your warm-up, as balance is a key component of bodybuilding.

1. Get ready for your dead lift. Place your arms by your sides and your feet together as you stand. Raise your right arm and your left leg simultaneously, then return both to their initial positions. After ten repetitions, swap, raising your left arm and leg. Also perform 10 repetitions of those.

2. Walk like a duck. Maintaining a straight back when squatting, take a slow step forward and never raise yourself up into a standing position. Repeat these steps three times around your room.

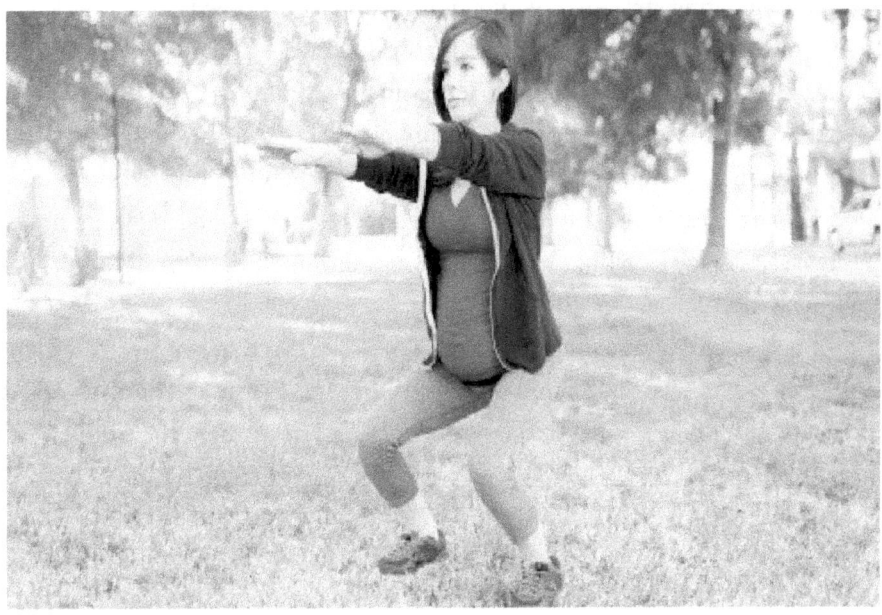

3. Include a little yoga. Lift your arms above your head while maintaining a leg-together stance. Raise your right leg and extend it in front of you for ten seconds. Lower it, then lower your left leg and repeat the action. Finish five leg lifts each.

Workouts for the Upper Body

Your back, shoulders, chest, and arms should be your main areas of concentration when it comes to building your upper body. Although these workouts are simple enough for novices to perform, they will help you develop a stronger upper body. Pushing and pulling are the main exercises for the upper body. We split these workouts up into those two categories.

Pull

1. Perform three sets of twelve dumbbell curls on each side. Start with a weighted dumbbell that you are comfortable with. 3 pounds, 5 pounds, or even 10 pounds could be the weight. Perform this workout on a bench or chair. Put one hand on the bench or chair seat and flatten your back. Keep your arm hanging straight at your side while using the other hand to hold the weight. Raise and bend your arm till your elbow lines up with your body's side. Reposition the arm after a brief moment of holding.

2. Perform three sets of twelve dumbbell curls. Position yourself with a dumbbell in each hand and your arms straight, keeping your feet shoulder-width apart. Pull both of your arms up in front of you, bending them at the elbows, as you are curling. Hold them for a moment, then straighten them out once more.

3. Employ a resistance stretch band to perform three sets of twelve weight pulls. Step on the stretch band and hold each end firmly in your hands. As with the dumbbells, keep your arms straight and bend them to curl up.

HOME EXERCISES FOR STRENGTH TRAINING

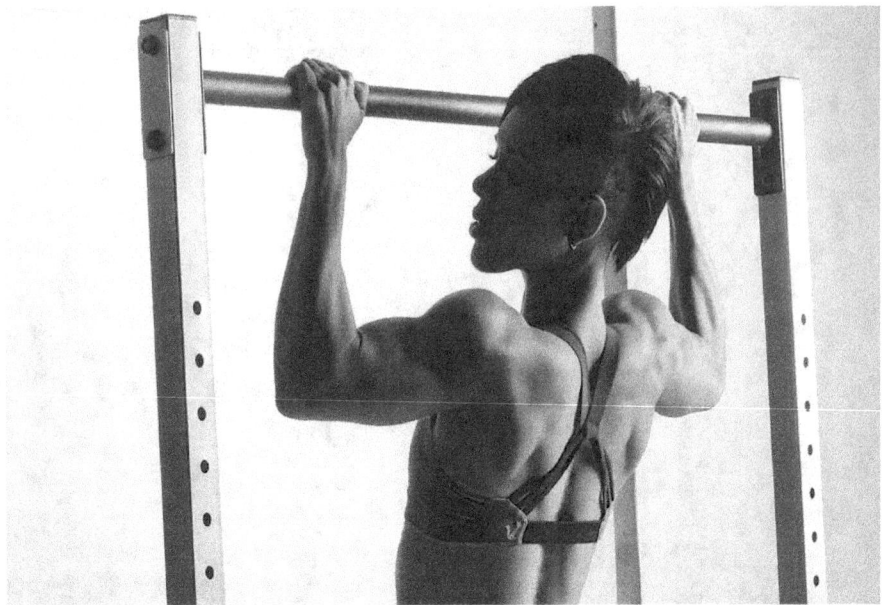

Pushing

1. Try three sets of ten push-ups. With your palms flat on the ground in front of you and spaced shoulder-width apart, drop to your knees. Lower your upper body toward the ground while maintaining a straight back and remaining on your knees. Push yourself back up as soon as your chin is almost in contact with the floor. Get off your knees and perform standard push-ups, keeping your knees off the ground, as your strength increases.

2. Execute twelve sets of trice extensions. Arms bent, place your dumbbells in your hands as you lie on your back. When your arms are nearly fully extended, push the dumbbells up and away from your body. Repeat after lowering them once more to your chest. Attempt to keep your elbows as near to your body as you can.

3. Perform twelve shoulder extensions in three sets. Position yourself with the dumbbells in your hands and your legs shoulder-width apart. The weights should be exactly at your shoulders as you bend your arms. Once your arms are nearly straight, push them past your head and up into the air. Reposition them so they are at your shoulders slowly.

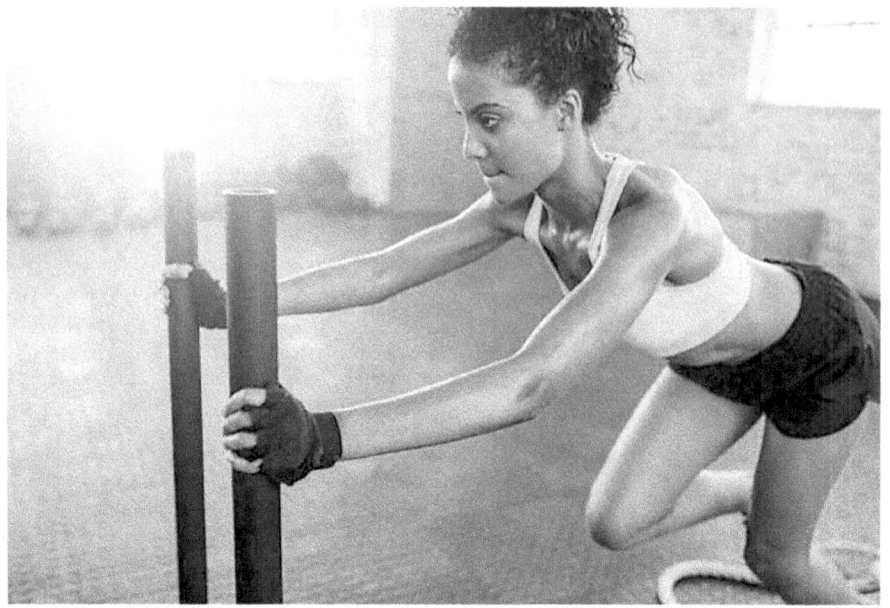

Core & Abdominal Exercises

Without a strong core, building your physique is impossible. Your lower back, glutes, and abdominal muscles make up your core. You'll gain the fundamental strength from these exercises, which will help you achieve better bodybuilding outcomes.

Exercises for the Abstinence

1. Perform ten hip lifts in three sets. While lying on the floor, raise your legs straight and fix your gaze on your toes. Put your arms at your sides on the ground and flex your feet. Raising your hips a few inches off the ground will cause your feet to point toward the ceiling without causing you to sway or move your body. Reposition your hips so that your lower back is on the ground.

2. Perform three sets of ten V-Ups. Place your arms at your sides and your legs straight out on the floor while you lie on your back. Once you get into a V stance, raise your head and shoulders simultaneously with your legs. Together with your legs, your arms should rise off the ground. Return to the floor by lowering yourself.

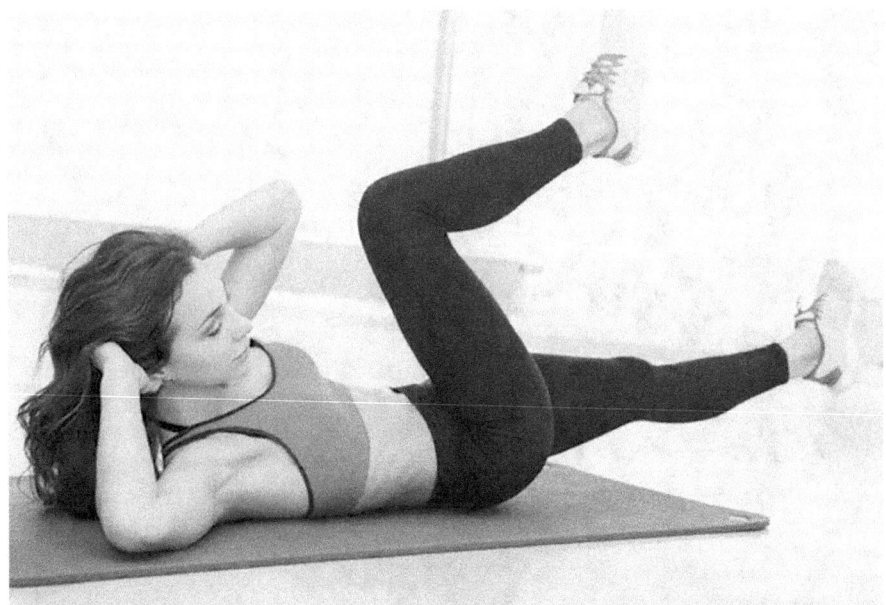

Core Workouts

Perform three sets of ten repetitions of the downward dog kick. Position yourself in an inverted V form by pressing your hips up and back while on all fours. Lift and maintain a straight leg as you kick your right behind you. Do ten, then move to the left leg and perform ten more.

2. For ten seconds or more, hold a plank three times. With your hands flat on the floor, your elbows bent, and your toes tucked beneath your feet, lie on your stomach. As you raise yourself into the plank position, make sure your back is flat and your arms are nearly straight (don't lock your elbows). Although many people find it more challenging, you can also maintain this position with your elbows on the floor.

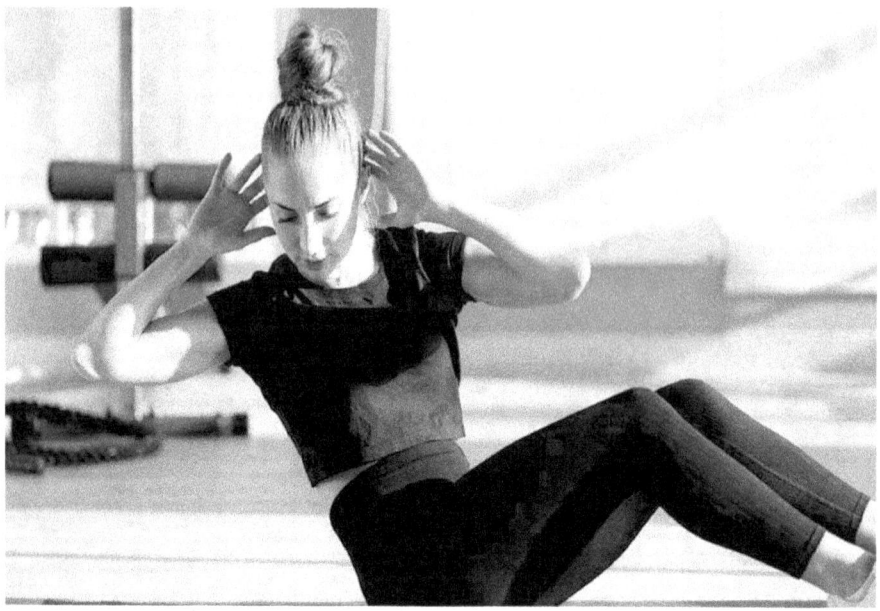

Glutei Exercises

1. Complete 16 hip thrusts in 3 sets. Position yourself on your back, knees bent, and spaced shoulder-width apart. Shoulders still on the ground, press your hips toward the ceiling. Once again, lower yourself to the floor after holding the position for three seconds.

2. Perform ten sets of leg kicks. With your hands and knees shoulder-width apart, go into a full crawl. Straighten and raise your right leg as high as you can behind you. The knee should be bent and brought back without touching the ground. Repeatedly kick. Kick the right leg first, then the left.

HOME EXERCISES FOR STRENGTH TRAINING

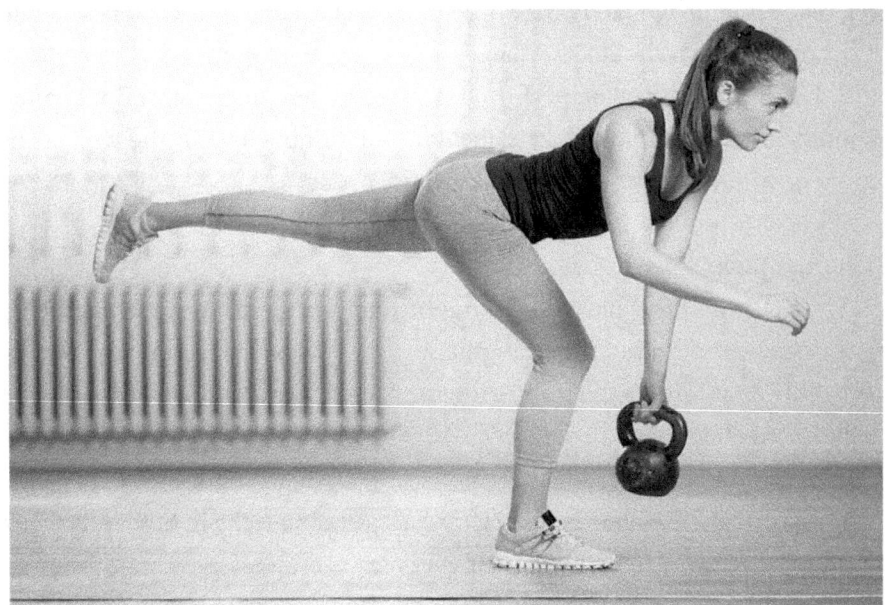

Workouts for the Lower Body

Strengthening your thighs, hamstrings, hips, and quadriceps is what you should aim for while working on your lower body. Increased muscle growth, balance, and range of motion are all benefits of these exercises.

Lower Body Exercises

1. Perform three sets of 12 squats. Place your hands on your hips and stand with your legs shoulder-width apart. With your back straight, lower your chest and slowly bend your knees to descend toward the earth. As much as possible, descend, but don't lose the ability to push yourself back up to a standing position.

2. Perform 10 weighted squats in 3 sets. Grasp a dumbbell or kettlebell in front of you using both hands. Lift the weight to your chest and bend your arms as you squat. Straightening out of the squat, lower the weight.

Lunges

1. Perform ten lunge steps in three sets. Step one foot in front of the other, bending both legs until your rear knee almost touches the floor and your front

leg reaches approximately ninety degrees. Make sure your back is straight. Legs one and two should alternate.

2. Holding your weight, perform three sets of ten lunge steps. Both hands should be used to hold one kettlebell or two dumbbells. Lift the weights in front of you to your chest as you finish your lunges.

Leaping Jacks

The majority of us have done jumping jacks since we were young. This is an excellent workout for strengthening the quads, glutes, and hip flexors. In addition, it targets the stabilizing muscles of the shoulders, hamstrings, calves, and abdomen.

This workout is excellent for increasing both strength and endurance simultaneously. Go ahead and perform 40 jumping jacks in three sets. This is an excellent way to wrap up your everyday exercise.

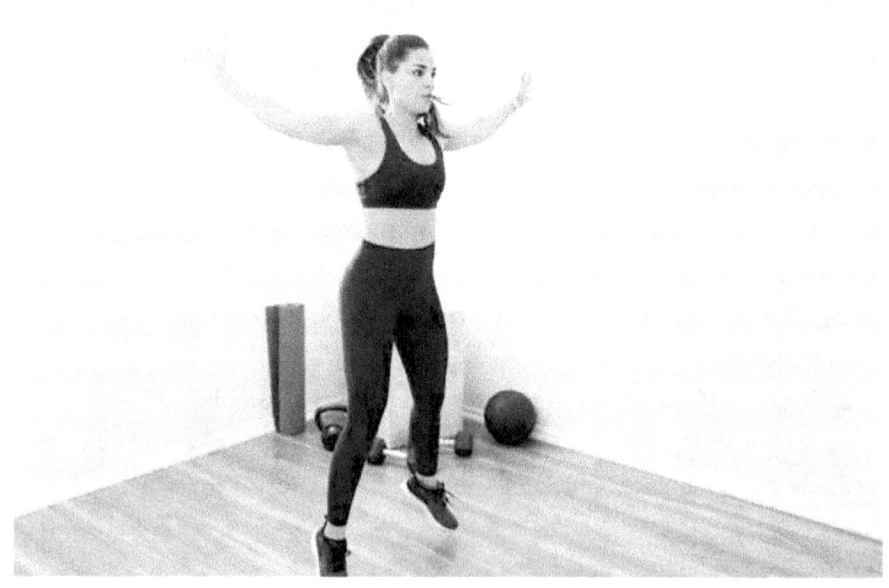

Extra Exercises for the Lower Body

1. Perform three sets of ten hip abductions. Using a chair or barre as support, stand with your legs together. While maintaining an erect posture, extend your right leg to the side. Release it to the earth. After ten reps on your right side, move on to your left leg. Your hips get stronger and more extended with this workout.

2. Perform three sets of ten hip stretches. Using a chair or barre as support, stand with your legs together. Keeping your back straight and your left leg straight, swing your right leg back behind you. Release it to the earth. After ten reps on your right side, move on to your left leg.

3. Complete 15 toe raises in three sets. Holding the back of a chair or a barre for support, stand with your legs together. As you raise yourself to your toes, you should feel the muscles in your calves contract. Return to the earth by lowering your body. Never take a longer than a few seconds to get back up on your toes after resting.

Example of a 7-Day Training Schedule

Considering your fitness regimen for entire weeks at a time is necessary now that you know what kinds of workouts you may combine with strength training routines at home. Make sure to concentrate on every aspect of strength training when you're organizing your schedule. Resting is also essential for the healing of your body and muscles. For those who are just starting out in bodybuilding, this sample 7-day schedule is a great starting point.

First Day: Lower Body

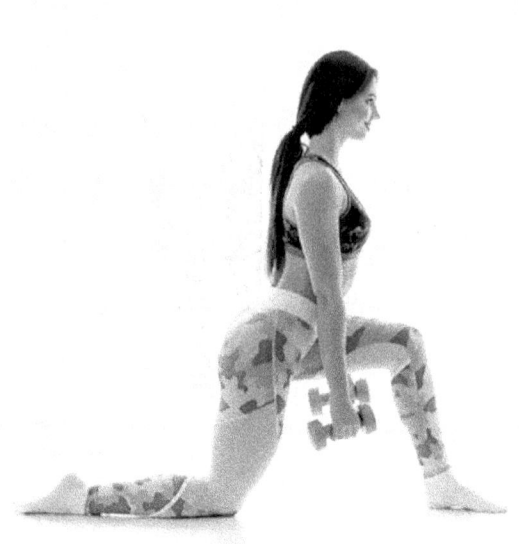

1. Warm up for ten minutes to begin. If you have a treadmill at home, use it to walk briskly around your area. Spend an additional five minutes warming up your legs and hips because it is a lower body workout. Perform 3 sets of skips and 3 sets of marches.

2. Perform three 12-squat sets.

3. Perform 10 lunge steps in 3 sets.

4. Perform three sets of ten hip abductions on each leg.

5. Perform three sets of ten hip extenders for each leg.

6. Practice the Warrior Pose. This is a yoga stance that tones the legs and lower back. With the toe facing forward, place your right foot at least three or four feet in front of you. To maintain your balance, extend and rotate your left leg as necessary. Allowing your front leg to bear the majority of your weight, raise your arms above your head and fix your gaze on your palms. After holding for at least 15 seconds, rotate so that your left leg is in front.

Day Two: Upper Body

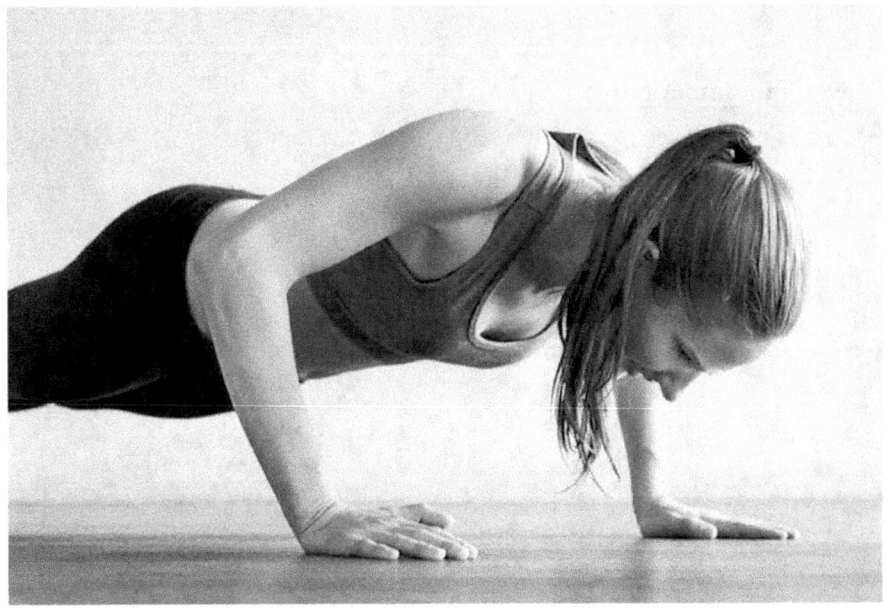

1. Warm up for ten minutes to begin. Stroll or run. Continue warming up your arms for 5 minutes by performing 3 sets of 10 arm circles.

2. Perform three sets of ten pushups.

3. Perform three sets of twelve resistance pulls using a stretch band.

4. Perform three sets of twelve arm raises. Let your arms dangle freely at your sides while you hold a dumbbell in each hand. Raise your arms until you can reach them above your head. Lower them gradually until they are at rest. Raise them one more. Maintain a straight arm posture.

5. Complete 3 more sets of 10 push-ups.

Day 3: Relaxation

Keep an eye on your nutrition during your day of rest. If you can, engage in some unstructured physical activity. At the park, chase your kids around, go swimming, or go for a stroll.

It's crucial to emphasize this in order to optimize the benefits of bodybuilding exercises: muscle growth does not happen during exercise. Rather, throughout the recovery period following an exercise, your muscles heal and expand. Because of this, bodybuilding requires consuming a balanced diet and getting enough sleep.

Day 4: Fundamentals

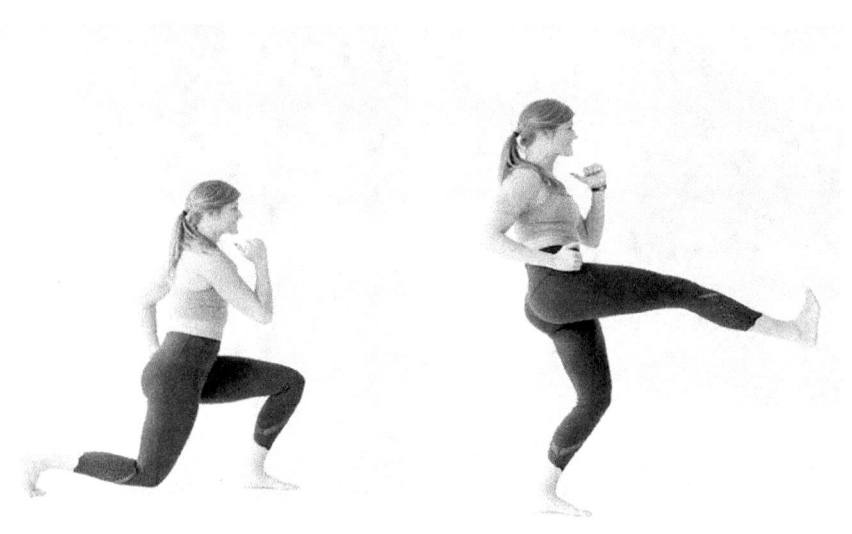

1. Jump rope or perform jumping jacks for ten minutes to warm up. You can even briskly walk or sprint in place. For an additional five minutes, practice neck rolls. To begin, nod affirmatively, then roll your head in full circles.

2. Perform ten sets of shoulder shrugs. Elevate your shoulders toward your ears while keeping your feet together. Reduce them gradually.

3. For ten seconds or longer, hold a plank.

4. Complete three sets of ten V-Ups.

5. Maintain a 10-second grip on another plank.

6. Complete 3 sets of 15 side bends. Place the soles of your feet shoulder-width apart. Lift the arm across your head as you bend to one side. Return to the center, lift your other arm over your head, and bend the other direction.

7. Maintain a 10-second grip on another plank.

Day Five: Lower Body

1. Start with a vigorous jog or 10-minute stroll to warm up. March and skip for five more minutes.

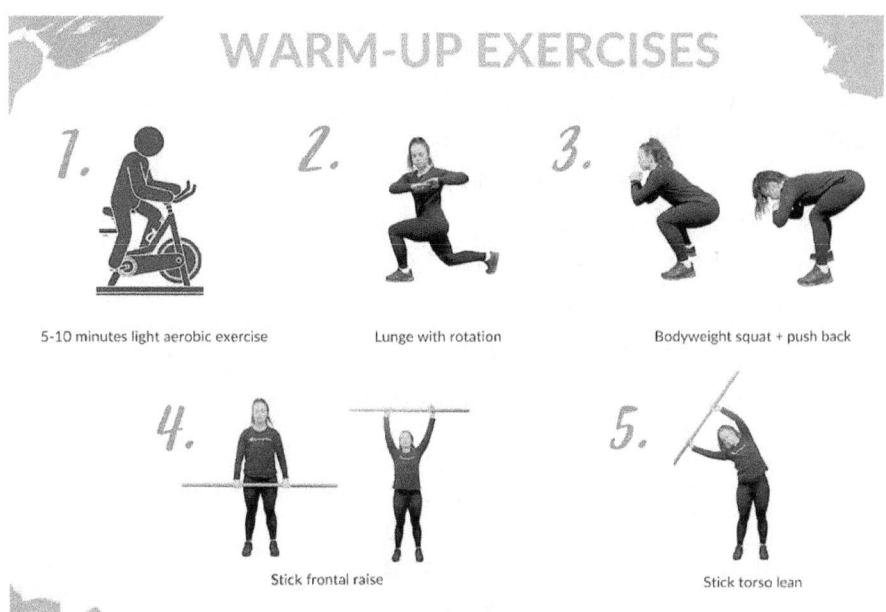

2. Complete 12 chair squats in 3 sets. This exercise is identical to a standard squat, only you will perform it while standing in front of a chair. After lowering yourself to almost the chair, raise yourself back up.

3. Complete 15 toe raises in three sets.

4. Perform three sets of twelve side leg lifts. Lie on your right side on the ground. Lean your legs apart while supporting your upper torso with your elbows. Elevate and descend your left leg while maintaining your right leg on the ground. Flip over and finish the opposite side as well.

5. Perform three sets of ten side lunges. Place your hands on your hips and stand with your feet together. Leap as deep as you can without falling as you take a big step to the right. Reposition yourself so that you are in the center. Go around to the left.

Day 6: Take a break

Particularly after another day of working out your lower body, you can be sore. Take a slow stroll to stretch out your healing muscles and give your body time to recuperate.

Day 7: Upper and Core Body

1. Walk or jog for ten minutes to warm up. Perform shoulder rolls, toe raises, and neck rolls for five minutes.
2. For ten seconds or longer, hold a plank.
3. Perform ten V-Ups in three sets of 3.
4. Perform 15 Hip Thrusts in three sets.
5. Perform three sets of ten hip lifts.
6. Perform three sets of ten pushups.

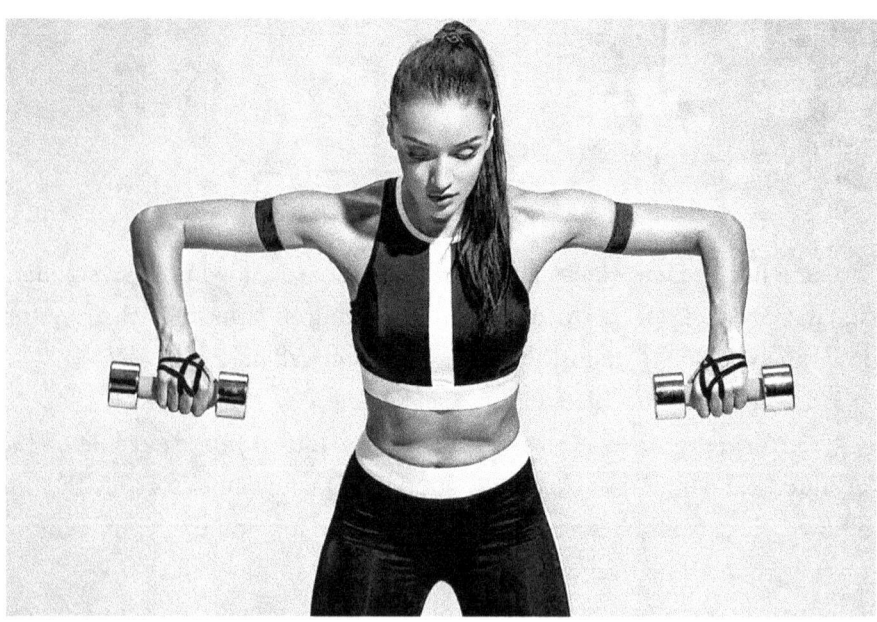

Strength Training Activities for the Home: Diverse

Avoiding boredom is crucial. When you use dumbbells, kettlebells, or other weights, you'll notice that the repetitions get easier and you can lift heavier weights as your strength and endurance increase. You should constantly be searching for fresh workouts to add to your regimen for strength training. The beginner-friendly activities in this book are designed to help you begin to comprehend the physical sensations in your body and the potential for personal development that you possess. Make sure you attempt some alternative exercises and learn some other ways to improve your body and increase your strength if you start to get bored or the routines start to grow dull. Even though strength training is your main priority right now rather than cardio, modest cardio routines are still appropriate. It improves your general physical fitness, leg strength, and heart health.

You can work out at home with these strength training exercises. You can join a gym to help you with your efforts when you're ready to move on to weight lifting machines. Learn these easy workouts for the time being so that you may lay a solid basis for your training regimen. When working out with a friend, some people discover that their results are higher. In order to make sure you're on track given your current skill level and your growth aspirations, review the strategy and the program if you choose to proceed with this.

3

What to Eat for Nutrition in Bodybuilding

How strength training and exercise result in muscle growth is one of the main questions in bodybuilding. Your muscle fibers are slightly ripped and injured when you perform strength or weight training. This activates a unique subset of cells called satellite cells, which are found in close proximity to the body's muscle cells. After multiplying, activated satellite cells merge with the injured muscle fibers to repair and strengthen them. Furthermore, the muscle cells' creation of new proteins is stimulated by the satellite cells. When combined, these processes increase the thickness and strength of the rebuilt muscles relative to their pre-workout state.

Your diet is a crucial factor to consider when starting a strength training program. Your body gets its fuel from the food you eat, which also supplies the nutrients required for muscle growth, repair, and maintenance. It's crucial to eat enough to support your optimum physical performance rather than going on a rigid diet and cutting back on meals and calories. Protein is the main component of a bodybuilding diet since it helps you create muscle and burn fat. It also helps you get stronger.

Concentrate on Protein

Your diet for bodybuilding will be centered around protein. The fuel for your cells is protein. It permits the maintenance and proliferation of your tissues, especially muscular tissue. In addition, your body utilizes protein to make hormones and to shield your blood, skin, and bones. Many of your body's activities slow down and become worse if you don't eat enough protein. Your bones could become more fragile, your skin and hair could become dull, and you would lose muscle. Increasing your protein intake when starting a strength training program is necessary because you are not only maintaining but also developing a strong and healthy physique.

Direct food sources are the best sources of protein. You are allowed to eat fish, eggs, and lean meats like beef, hog, and turkey. In addition, legumes like beans and tofu, as well as nuts and seeds, provide protein. Protein bars, powders, and shakes are added to diets by certain individuals. This is an excellent method to incorporate the beneficial protein elements into your diet and give yourself a burst of energy. But in order to prevent hunger, you should make an effort to consume as much genuine protein as you can. A healthy, high-protein breakfast will provide you with a solid foundation to build upon and provide you with the energy you need to get through your exercises and the rest of the day. Start your day with a plate of eggs.

There are additional benefits to including protein in your diet when gaining muscle. Because you'll feel fuller, you won't be as prone to reach for unhealthy snacks during the day. Because it improves your metabolism, the protein will also aid in your increased ability to burn fat. You'll have extra energy since your body will turn the protein into glucose. Reduced carbohydrate and increased protein diets have also been shown to help with weight loss and improve heart health.

There are lipids included in many protein sources. It's nothing to worry about too much. Particularly when you're gaining muscle, your body also needs the fat. You're doing your body a favor if you're consuming foods high in healthy fats, such nuts, fish, and oils.

Nutrition Before and After Exercise

Your performance will be greatly impacted by the foods you consume both before and after strength training sessions. In order to have the energy necessary to lift weights and develop your physique, have some high-quality carbohydrates and protein before working out. Try some whole grain oats topped with nuts and berries, or scrambled eggs over a slice of high-fiber bread if you enjoy working out in the morning. It's a good idea to consume brown rice or pasta about an hour before beginning strength training if you work out in the afternoon or evening.

You must consume some protein to aid in the recovery of your muscles after working out. Eat a piece of fish or some grilled chicken. To nourish and rebuild your muscles in the absence of a full meal, consider consuming a protein smoothie or bar. Avoid eating anything high on the glycemic index and make sure you drink enough of water. They will sap your vitality and make you feel exhausted during your strength training session. It's not a good idea to eat empty carbs, which come from sugars and junk food, before or after doing exercise.

Healthy Consumption

A diet rich in protein and healthy carbohydrates is the norm for most bodybuilders who achieve success. Processed foods can only make you slower and cause weight gain because they are high in sugar, added fats, and salt. When gaining weight for bodybuilding, it's important to ensure that you're gaining healthy, lean muscle rather than fat. A nutritious, well-balanced diet that works well with a strength training program is how to achieve that.

The best diet is one that is clean. Pick proteins, vitamins, and minerals that are abundant in local, sustainable sources and that will help you gain muscle. Include eggs, salmon, chicken, turkey, and lean meat in your meals. Use important carbohydrates like brown rice, healthy grain bread, pasta, and sweet potatoes to complement that protein. In order to maintain your body healthy and improve your intake of fiber, include some seasonal fruits and leafy green vegetables. Choose helpful probiotic foods like yogurt and almonds and seeds as your snack options. By supporting all of the muscle building you're attempting to achieve, clean eating can help with your bodybuilding nutrition. Your body will feel well-fed and prepared for action. There are twenty tasty and healthful clean eating recipes in Chapter 4.

Avoid following fad diets. Even while reducing weight may be one of your fitness objectives, you shouldn't drastically cut back on your caloric consumption. Your body won't be able to grow stronger and more muscular if you do that. Consider the kinds of food you're selecting rather than just keeping track of calories. It will matter far more what you eat than how many calories or grams of fat are in it.

Workouts are more important than your diet during bodybuilding. Lifting weights consistently and hard is the best approach to gain muscle. You'll have to make time for lifting heavier weights and working out more frequently. The outcomes you can attain when you pair that with the appropriate diet will astound you.

4

Recipes for Healthful Eating

Most diet programs focus on one or more food groups, calories, or the proportion of fat to protein in the diet. It's much easier to eat clean. Eating as naturally as possible can be summed up as clean eating. Eat as many things as possible in their original state; that is the general philosophy behind it. This entails choosing raw or less processed meals. Except insofar as they are desired, you are not specifically excluding or adding any meals. There's no reason to stress over protein requirements, calorie counts, or nightshade vegetable avoidance.

Green Eggs for Breakfast
Double the yield.
Ingredients list:
four eggs
two cups of young spinach leaves
One diced stalk of celery, one diced zucchini, and one-half cup diced green bell pepper
A single tablespoon of almond milk
A single spoonful of olive oil
Add salt and pepper to taste.

Instructions:

1. In a skillet, heat the oil over medium heat. Cook for three minutes after adding the celery, zucchini, and green pepper.

2. After adding the spinach, simmer it until it starts to wilt.

3. After adding the almond milk, beat the eggs with a fork or whisk. Transfer all of the vegetables into the skillet and scramble.

4. Add a dash of pepper and salt.

Information about Nutrition (Per Serving)

Calorie count: 229

5.4 g of saturated fat and 17.8 g of total fat

6.3 grams of carbs

1.9 grams of fiber

3.5 grams of sugar

Protein: 13.1%

Four dishes of breakfast casserole

Ingredients list:

Four red potatoes, chopped and peeled

A cup of peeled and chopped eggplant and a cup of peeled and chopped butternut squash

Four garlic cloves

One red bell pepper, chopped; one green bell pepper, chopped; one sliced red onion

Two cups broccoli

four tsp of olive oil

One stem of fresh rosemary

Four new leaves of basil

Add salt and pepper to taste.

Guidelines:

Warm up your oven to 375 degrees Fahrenheit. Stir until everything is well blended after adding the olive oil.

2. Bake for 40 minutes, or until the veggies are bubbling and tender.

Data on Nutrition (Per Serving)

Calories : 328
Fat : 14.6 g
Sat Fat : 2.1 g
Carbohydrates : 47.5 g
Fiber : 7.6 g
Sugar : 6.9 g
Protein : 6.7 g

Produce Your Own Granola

- 6 servings are produced.
- Ingredients list:
- one cup of almonds
- one cup cashews
- ½ cup walnuts
- Half a cup of raisins
- one cup of oats
- 1/4 cup of coconut shreds
- One-fourth cup of sunflower seeds
- One-half cup of pine nuts
- Three tsp of cinnamon
- two cups of almond milk

Instructions

1. Combine all of the dry ingredients in a mixer until well blended.
2. Transfer to four bowls, and then top each with ½ cup almond milk.

Nutritional Information (Per Serving)

Calories : 471
Fat : 33.5 g
Sat Fat : 5.5 g
Carbohydrates : 36.4 g
Fiber : 6.8 g

Sugar : 11.9 g
Protein : 13.3 g
Sodium : 55 mg

Smoothie with Berries Explosion

Produced 1 serving; Ingredients:

½ cup of blueberries

1/4 cup of strawberries

Half a cup of raspberries

One-half cup blackberries

One-half banana

A single cup of almond milk

Half a cup of ice

Guidelines:

1. Put all the ingredients into your blender and blend on high for 30 seconds.

Nutritional Information (Per Serving)

Calories: 240

Fat: 3.9 g

Sat Fat: 0.1 g

Carbohydrates: 51.8 g

Fiber: 12.5 g

Sugar: 30.2 g

Protein: 4.4 g

Sodium: 147 mg

Yield: 8 serves of carrot bread Ingredients list:

Two cups of almond flour

One-tspn baking powder

One tablespoon of seeds from cumin

To taste, add salt.

Three huge eggs

Two teaspoons of olive oil

One-tspn apple cider vinegar

Three cups of peeled and grated carrots

½ teaspoon finely grated, freshly peeled ginger

A quarter cup of raisins

Instructions:

1. Set the oven's temperature to 350 degrees Fahrenheit.
2. Line a loaf pan with baking parchment.
3. Place the almond flour, baking powder, cumin seeds, and salt in a big bowl and well stir.
4. Transfer the eggs, vinegar, and olive oil to a different bowl and mix everything together thoroughly.
5. Mix the egg mixture thoroughly with the flour mixture after adding it.
6. Add the raisins, carrot, and ginger and fold gently.
7. Spoon mixture into loaf pan that has been prepared.
8. Bake for approximately one hour, or until a toothpick inserted in the middle comes out clean.

Nutritional Information (Per Serving)

Calories: 133

Fat: 8.9 g

Sat Fat: 1.3 g

Carbohydrates: 10 g

Fiber: 2 g

Sugar: 4.9 g

Protein: 4.5 g

Southwest Chicken Wrap for lunch; yields 1 serve

Ingredients list:

One tortilla made of whole wheat

Half a cup of shredded carrots and six ounces of cooked chicken

Cut ¼ cup red bell pepper and boil ¼ cup black beans

Two avocado slices

one tsp of dehydrated cilantro

One teaspoon of red pepper flakes

Lime juice, ½ of it

Follow these instructions:

1. Place the chicken pieces on the tortilla, then top with avocado, beans, pepper, and carrots.

2. Drizzle the whole dish with lime juice, and garnish with cilantro and red pepper flakes. Twist to form a wrap.

Nutritional Information (Per Serving)

Calories: 565

Fat: 15.9 g

Sat Fat: 3.4 g

Carbohydrates: 47.2 g

Fiber: 13.6 g

Sugar: 5.6 g

Protein: 60 g

Sodium: 260 mg

Yield: 1 serving of chicken and rice bowl Ingredients list:

Half a cup of cooked brown rice

¼ cup of cooked chicken and ¼ cup of chopped tomatoes

1/4 cup of cooked corn

Half a cup of black beans boiled

One lime

Add salt and pepper to taste.

Instructions:

1. Add the black beans, corn, and chicken to the brown rice and mix everything together.

2. Add pepper, salt, and fresh tomatoes on top. Pour lime juice over it.

Nutritional Information (Per Serving)
Calories: 299
Fat: 3.5 g
Sat Fat: 0.8 g
Carbohydrates: 42.3 g
Fiber: 7.7 g
Sugar: 3.6 g
Protein: 27.7 g

Double the amount of tuna salad
Ingredients list:
four cups of lettuce
One can of tuna submerged in water
A tsp of olive oil
one tsp freshly squeezed lemon juice
1/4 cup sliced red bell pepper, 1/4 cup minced kalamata olives, and 1/4 cup sun-dried tomatoes
one celery stalk, diced
One tsp. of dried oregano
Steps to follow:
1. Clean, pat dry, and arrange lettuce on a platter to make a bed.
2. Combine the tuna, oregano, lemon juice, and olive oil in a bowl. Mix everything together after adding the veggies.
3. Spoon the tuna mixture onto the bed of lettuce and season with salt and pepper.
4. You can optionally drizzle with a little extra olive oil.

Nutritional Information (Per Serving)
Calories: 232
Fat: 9.3 g
Sat Fat: 1.6 g
Carbohydrates: 16 g
Fiber: 4.3 g

Sugar: 7.9 g
Protein: 23.5 g
Sodium: 633 mg

Sweet potatoes with garlic

Produced 1 serving; Ingredients:
One medium sweet potato, peeled and sliced into round, thin pieces
A tsp of olive oil
Add salt and pepper to taste.
1 smashed garlic clove
One teaspoon of parsley, cut finely
1/2 grated orange peel

Directions:

1. Set oven temperature to 400 degrees Fahrenheit.
2. Combine the oil, salt, pepper, and sweet potato in a bowl.
3. Lay out the potato slices on a sizable baking sheet and brush with cooking spray. Once the potato slice is golden brown, roast it for an additional 10 minutes after flipping it over.
4. Take out the potato slices, then stack them in a basin.
5. In a bowl, combine the parsley, lemon rind, and crushed garlic. Sprinkle this mixture over the sweet potato slices. Warm up and serve.

Nutritional Information (Per Serving)

Calories: 149
Fat: 4.9 g
Sat Fat: 0.7 g
Carbohydrates: 25.2 g
Fiber: 4.1 g
Sugar: 7.4 g
Protein: 2.6 g

Yield: 6 serves of Turkey and Bean Chili

Ingredients list:

Two pounds of pounded turkey breast, three cloves of garlic, one minced red onion, one diced green bell pepper, and two tablespoons of olive oil

Six raw tomatoes, peeled and diced; six ounces tomato paste

Four teaspoons of ground cumin, one cup of washed red kidney beans, one cup of rinsed black beans, and one cup of rinsed garbanzo beans

one tsp finely ground coriander

Two tsp of chili powder

One cup of water

1/4 teaspoon of salt

Instructions:

1. In a large soup pot, sauté turkey over medium heat for about 10 minutes, or until browned. Chili powder, coriander, and cumin should be added.

2. After removing the turkey from the pot, cover it with olive oil. Add the bell pepper, onion, and garlic and cook until tender.

3. Add salt and the tomatoes. Simmer the tomatoes for ten minutes or so. Next, put the meat back in the pot along with the beans and tomato paste.

4. Combine all of the ingredients by stirring. Add water to cover. Simmer for thirty minutes with a lid on.

Nutritional Information (Per Serving)

Calories: 745

Fat: 20.4 g

Sat Fat: 4.4 g

Carbohydrates: 76.2 g

Fiber: 20 g

Sugar: 13.7 g

Protein: 67.6 g

Sodium: 758 mg

Munchies

Cracked Egg Whites

Produces twelve servings.

Ingredients: ½ cup rinsed capers; ½ cup minced olives; ¼ cup sliced red bell pepper; 6 hardboiled and peeled eggs;

A single spoonful of olive oil

Add salt and pepper to taste.

Guidelines:

1. Split the eggs lengthwise, removing the yolks.
2. Add a little salt and pepper to the egg whites.
3. Add the olives, red pepper, and olive oil to a small bowl and use a fork to crush the capers. Combine and mix. Scoop the mixture into the egg whites' holes.

Nutritional Information (Per Serving)

Calories: 49

Fat: 4 g

Sat Fat: 0.9 g

Carbohydrates: 0.9 g

Fiber: 0.3 g

Sugar: 0.3 g

Protein: 2.9 g

Pasta Kababs

Four servings are produced.

Ingredients list:

Chop two celery stalks into big pieces.

One cup of button mushrooms, white

One cup of chilled cubed chicken

One cup heirloom carrots

one cup of olives

Cut one red pepper into pieces.

Cut one green pepper into pieces.

Cups of cauliflower florets and a half cup of olive oil

one tablespoon of oregano

Directions: Add salt and pepper to taste.

1. Combine all the ingredients in a bowl, stir to combine, and drizzle with olive oil.
2. Take a 30-minute break.
3. Arrange the food in stacks on skewers.

Nutritional Information (Per Serving)

Calories: 244
Fat: 17.6 g
Sat Fat: 2.6 g
Carbohydrates: 11.4 g
Fiber: 4.3 g
Sugar: 4.1 g
Protein: 13.2 g

Roasted Nuts and Seeds

Produced 15 servings.
Ingredients list:
one cup of almonds
one cup of walnuts
1 cup almonds
One cup of peanuts
Pumpkin seeds: ½ cup; sunflower seeds: ¼ cup
One-half cup of pine nuts
A pair of fresh rosemary sprigs
Six new sage leaves
One tsp cayenne pepper
A single spoonful of olive oil

Directions: Add salt and pepper to taste.

1. Preheat the oven to 400 degrees Fahrenheit.

2. Cover a baking sheet with the nuts and seeds. Add the salt, pepper, cayenne, and olive oil on top. Incorporate the sage and rosemary.

3. Bake for roughly twenty minutes.

4. Take out and let it settle.

Nutritional Information (Per Serving)

Calories: 228

Fat: 20.9 g

Sat Fat: 2.1 g

Carbohydrates: 6 g

Fiber: 3.1 g

Sugar: 1.1 g

Protein: 8.2 g

Four serves of the cinnamon fruit salad

Ingredients list:

One cup blueberries and two bananas, cut.

One-cup sliced strawberries and one-cup red grapes

one cup of green grapes

Two cups cubed watermelon and one cored, peeled, and diced apple

Two tsp freshly squeezed lemon juice

one spoonful of cinnamon

Instructions:

1. In a large bowl, combine all the fruits and stir. After all the fruits are combined, squeeze the lemon juice over them.

2. To ensure that all of the tastes meld, let the fruits chill for at least half an hour.

3. Top with a sprinkle of cinnamon and serve.

Nutritional Information (Per Serving)

Calories: 186

Fat: 0.8 g

Sat Fat: 0.2 g
Carbohydrates: 47.5 g
Fiber: 6.2 g
Sugar: 33.1 g
Protein: 2.3 g
Sodium: 6 mg

Excellent Green Juice

Produced 1 serving; Ingredients:
½ avocado
One-half cucumber
One cup of spinach
¼ cup fresh mint leaves; one celery stalk
one tsp finely grated ginger, just off the vine
One cup of water
Half a cup of ice

Instructions:

1. Put all the ingredients in a blender and process until the ice is broken up and the vegetables are well-combined.

Information about Nutrition (Per Serving)

Calories: 242
Fat: 20.1 g
Sat Fat: 4.3 g
Carbohydrates: 16.2 g
Fiber: 9.8 g
Sugar: 2.2 g
Protein: 4.3 g
Sodium: 52 mg

Sweet and Sour Salmon for Dinner

Four servings are produced.

Ingredients list:

2 tablespoons finely chopped scallions and ¾ teaspoon minced fresh ginger root

One tsp finely chopped garlic

Two teaspoons of olive oil

Balsamic vinegar, two tablespoons

one tablespoon of honey

one-half teaspoon of crushed red pepper flakes

To taste, add salt.

Four 6-ounce salmon fillets

Steps to follow:

1. Combine all ingredients except salmon fillets in a big bowl.
2. Add the salmon and generously drizzle with marinade. For around eight hours, cover and chill the mixture, tossing from time to time.
3. Turn the heat up to medium-high on the grill.
4. Coat the grill grate in oil. Lay the salmon fillets 5 inches away from the heat source on the grill grate.
5. Cook the salmon fillets for five to ten minutes on the grill, turning them once around the halfway point or until the desired doneness.

Nutritional Information (Per Serving)

Calories: 308

Fat: 17.6 g

Sat Fat: 2.5 g

Carbohydrates: 5.5 g

Fiber: 0.2 g

Sugar: 4.5 g

Protein: 33.2 g

Cilantro Lime Shrimp

Four servings are produced.

Ingredients list:

One pound of tiny to medium-sized peeled and deveined shrimp

Two tomatoes, peeled and diced

Two limes

1/4 cup of raw cilantro

A quarter cup of olive oil

Add salt and pepper to taste.

Guidelines:

1. Warm the oven to 375 degrees Fahrenheit. In a bowl, toss the shrimp and tomatoes, then drizzle with olive oil.

2. Transfer to a baking dish and pour lime juice over top. Season with the salt, pepper, and cilantro.

3. Simmer for 20 minutes, or until the shrimp turn pink.

Nutritional Information (Per Serving)

Calories: 242

Fat: 14 g

Sat Fat: 2.2 g

Carbohydrates: 6 g

Fiber: 1.7 g

Sugar: 2.2 g

Protein: 24.5 g

Four servings of ginger steak

Ingredients list:

Eight smashed garlic cloves

two teaspoons of freshly sliced, raw ginger

one tablespoon of honey

A quarter cup of olive oil

Add salt and pepper to taste.

Trimmed 1½ pounds of flank steak

Guidelines:

1. Combine all the ingredients, excluding the steak, in a big sealable bag.
2. Include the meat and generously cover with marinade.
3. After sealing the bag, place it in the fridge to marinate for roughly a day.
4. Take out of the refrigerator and let the steak sit at room temperature for about fifteen minutes.
5. Place a grill pan on medium-high heat that has been lightly oiled. After removing the extra marinade from the steak, put it in a grill pan.
6. Cook until done, about 6 to 8 minutes on each side.
7. Take out of the grill pan and let it cool for ten minutes before slicing.
8. Cut into appropriate serving slices with a sharp knife and serve.

Nutritional Information (Per Serving)

Calories: 471
Fat: 37.9 g
Sat Fat: 1.8 g
Carbohydrates: 7 g
Fiber: 0.3 g
Sugar: 4.4 g
Protein: 24.4 g

Mustard-Sauerried Chicken

Produces 1 serving.
Ingredients list:
One-half tablespoon of olive oil
Two skinned, halved, and boneless chicken breasts
A dash of salt and a pinch of black pepper
Half a cup of chicken broth
A single spoonful of Dijon mustard
one tsp of butter
1 tsp finely chopped parsley

Directions:

1. Set oven temperature to 450 degrees Fahrenheit.

2. Dredge the chicken in the oil after seasoning it with salt and pepper. Transfer the chicken to an ovenproof pan and bake for approximately ten minutes, or until it has a browned appearance.

3. After the chicken is browned on one side, flip it over and continue cooking. Take the chicken out of the pan.

4. Add the chicken broth to the pan and heat it over medium-high heat until it becomes thick. Stir in the parsley, butter, and mustard.

5. Drizzle the chicken with the mustard sauce and present it hot.

Information about Nutrition (Per Serving)

Calories: 414
Fat: 21.4 g
Sat Fat: 5.4 g
Carbohydrates: 1.2 g
Fiber: 0.6 g
Sugar: 0.3 g
Protein: 52.1 g
Sodium: 1251 mg

Six serves of the curry with meatballs

Ingredients: 1 cup meatball mix

Lean ground turkey, one pound

Two beaten eggs

3 tablespoons finely chopped red onion; ¼ cup finely chopped fresh basil leaves; ¼ teaspoon finely chopped fresh ginger

four finely sliced cloves of garlic

One jalapeño jalapeno, chopped and seeded

A single tablespoon of pasted red curry

A tsp of fish sauce

two tsp of coconut oil

To taste, add salt.

For Curry:

One jalapeño pepper, seeded and diced; one red onion; four minced garlic cloves; and one ½ teaspoon of fresh ginger

two tsp red curry paste

One can (14 oz) of coconut milk

Two tsp freshly squeezed lime juice

Add salt and pepper to taste.

Directions:

The first step in making meatballs is to combine all the ingredients, excluding the oil, in a big bowl and mix everything together thoroughly. From the mixture, form tiny balls.

2. Melt coconut oil over medium heat in a big skillet. When the meatballs are golden brown on both sides, add them and simmer for 3 to 5 minutes. Once in a bowl, transfer the meatballs.

3. Sauté an onion for three minutes in the same skillet with a dash of salt.

4. Add the jalapeño, ginger, and garlic; sauté for one minute.

5. After adding the curry paste, cook for one minute.

6. After adding the meatballs and coconut milk, boil gently. For around ten minutes, simmer with a lid on on low heat.

7. Drizzle some lime juice over top and serve.

Nutritional Information (Per Serving)

Calories: 370

Fat: 29.5 g

Sat Fat: 20.8 g

Carbohydrates: 9.8 g

Fiber: 2.2 g

Sugar: 3.7 g

Protein: 19 g

5

Advice for Novices on Strength Training

It makes sense to get excited when you decide to start a strength training program. But it's crucial to pace yourself. Avoid pushing yourself too hard during your early sessions to the point of burnout or injury. These novice strength training suggestions will enable you to dedicate your time and attention to the exercise without setting unattainable goals for yourself.

First tip: Go at your own speed

There is no one to compete with when you first start out—not even yourself, even if you manage to make your way onto the competitive circuit. Working at your own pace and allowing yourself to get better over time is the aim. Comparing oneself to weightlifters who have been doing it for years or attempting to outdo a workout partner who also engages in strength training is pointless.

Remember who you are and what you want to achieve. Begin cautiously and with the quantity of exercises that you find manageable. You will most likely become discouraged, sore, and unable to continue if you declare that you will lift weights for two hours a day, seven days a week. Make modest, doable objectives. Start with a small weight or perhaps only two days a week. Start at a slower tempo and see if you can increase it.

Second Tip: Gradually Up the Intensity

Increase your intensity gradually when you've found a comfortable and sustainable pace. As you start to feel more comfortable lifting, go from a 10-pound weight to a 15-pound weight and continuing adding more. Apply the same principle to your repeats. Lift eight times at first, then ten, twelve, and finally fifteen. You'll discover your emotional state and the maximum amount of weight your muscles can support. In addition to preventing injuries, going cautiously will prevent you from giving up if you try to improve too quickly. Be patient and have faith in your body. Strength training is a long-term fitness program, not a sprint. Each two weeks, raise your weight.

Point Three: Pay Attention to Free Weights

Depending on the gym you go, you may be in awe of the intricate machinery and expensive machines. But keep in mind that using free weights—which you can use at home—is the ideal method to begin a strength training program. When you're stronger and ready for a more challenging workout, you can progress to the machines from barbells and dumbbells, which will help you develop a strong foundation of lean muscle mass. Get yourself some free weights that come in different sizes and weight ranges so you can lift things no matter where you are.

Fourth Tip: Take a Break

A lot of novices are so enthusiastic about their goals that they want to work out every day. Your body needs rest, though, and your muscles will take advantage of these days off to heal and rebuild themselves so you can work out again soon. Separate the muscle parts such that one day you work on your legs and the following day your arms and chest. Make an effort to follow a schedule for three or four days a week. Your body won't feel overly sore and you won't run the danger of injury, but this will give you enough of a plan to get used to doing out every other day.

Tip 5: Acquire Form Knowledge

Consider hiring a personal trainer or teaming up with someone who knows the proper form for lifting if you're unsure about either of these things. It will be difficult for you to break poor habits if, as a novice, you pick up bad skills. It could be necessary for you to continue at a reduced weight for a while until you are able to achieve and sustain the proper form. As you advance, though, it will be well worth it.

Tip 6: Give priority to safety

When working out, try to find a companion who can identify you, particularly when doing large lifts. When lifting weight that you have never lifted before, put on a safety belt and don't be embarrassed to ask for assistance. Bodybuilders with expertise can teach beginners a lot, and most of them are happy to share their knowledge and insights. To protect their hands, some bodybuilders use gloves. Exercise with caution and take all the necessary safety precautions.

Tip 7. Keep an Eye on Your Nutrition

You already know that diet plays a big part in how well you lift. Consume enough of protein, avoid junk food, and drink plenty of water before, during, and after workouts. Eat enough to sustain the quantity of energy you must expend throughout your weightlifting sessions, without restricting your calorie intake.

Tip 8. Try Compound Moves as a

At first, keep things straightforward. Keep your exercise routine simple. Rather, focus on the fundamentals. Squats, deadlifts, bench presses, and shoulder lifts should all be performed once a week. After you've mastered the fundamentals, build on your momentum with additional lifts that target the specific muscle groups you need to strengthen.

Tip 9: Adhere to Your Plan

Maintain your regimen once you've established it. Nothing else will produce the kind of outcomes that consistency will. You're getting a good workout in as long as you make time for each muscle group each week and feel that you've pushed yourself without going too far.

Tip 10: Adopt a Comprehensive View

Good general health is necessary for strength training. Don't let drugs, alcohol, or smoking ruin your plans. Aim for a healthy sleep schedule each night and develop stress management skills. Lifting weights is not the only thing you need to do to have an amazing body. It demands dedication to general health.

These ten strength training pointers for novices will increase your chances of developing a stronger physique. As you follow them, determine what is most effective for you. It's going to boost your bodybuilding success rate and results.

In conclusion

Women can benefit greatly from strength training in many ways. It is customizable based on your exercise level and daily routine. You'll be shocked at how rapidly you develop your capabilities when you start with modest weights and a few repetitions. With this book, I intend to burn fat and calories and help you develop a toned, slender figure.

Lastly, let me express my gratitude for having read my book. Please take a moment to write a review and share your opinions about the book on Amazon if you liked it. I would be really grateful for that!

6

Yoga for Novices

Simple Yoga Poses to Help You Relax,
Reduce Weight, and Boost Your Body's Strength

An Overview of Yoga

Yoga is a type of relaxation that balances the spirit, mind, and body. Through a sequence of breathing and stretching exercises, practitioners are able to reestablish a connection with both the environment and themselves. The origins of yoga disciplines can be traced back to ancient India as a collection of mental, spiritual, and physical disciplines. Actually, one of the six orthodox schools of Hindu philosophical traditions is this well-liked method of physical activity and stress-relief. Millions of people practice and love yoga today all around the world. Along with techniques and approaches deeply ingrained in Buddhism, Jainism, and of course Hinduism, there are also a variety of yoga schools.

Fundamentals of Yoga

Each and every yoga practitioner follows their own unique set of objectives, values, and tenets. But there are a few elements that all diverse styles and levels of yoga have in common. Among those principles is relaxation. There isn't any high impact running, jumping, or lifting like there is with other forms of exercise. You should concentrate on relaxing your body, mind, and soul. It takes effort to get your muscles to relax rather than tense up. You'll discover how to teach your body to unwind and maintain its flexibility.

Proper breathing is another principle. Yoga is a spiritual and ascetic discipline practiced by Hindus that teaches practitioners how to control and regulate their breath. The latter is crucial for opening your mind's eye, properly interacting with your ideas, and lowering daily stress, worry, and tension.

Another important aspect of yoga is nutrition, which is one of the reasons it helps so much with weight loss. In an attempt to maintain equilibrium in both your life and spirit, you will become aware of the nourishment you are giving your body. The idea is to fuel your body and mind with wholesome, freshly prepared foods. A serious yoga practice requires a light and strong body, and you'll get there faster if you're eating healthfully. Lastly, a key component of yoga is meditation. Using this method, mental clutter is removed from the mind and the body and soul are reunited as a single, harmonious whole.

A Synopsis of Yoga's History

The real roots of yoga have been debated, but most practitioners believe it began in India around 3000 B.C. This is the location of the Indus Valley's stone carvings depicting yoga practitioners. These pictures depict the initial yoga positions and techniques, which date back millennia before any modern, current, or social improvements were made. Yoga was and continues to be a vital means of ensuring soul and heart balance. Achieving heavenly enlightenment is the goal of every "yogi"—practitioner, disciple, teacher, or guru. This is essentially the recognition of a greater force, which to some may be nature or the celestial bodies, and to others may be God.

The Yoga Sutra's Eight Paths

The Yoga Sutra by Patanjali contains the eight limbs of yoga. These fundamental principles, known as ashtanga, are meant to assist practitioners in leading meaningful and purposeful lives. These limbs impart good morality, ethics, and self-discipline as a route to heavenly enlightenment. In a similar vein, they assist us in recognizing and addressing the spiritual facets of our nature and existence—all the while promoting better health and longer lifespans. According to Patanjali, yoga has eight limbs:

Yo
Yama is the initial branch of yoga. This discipline aids in helping us concentrate on our actions and the proper way to behave in daily life. It also imparts knowledge on our moral principles and sense of integrity. The Yamas, also known as the Golden Rule, are intended to be universal guidelines. "Do unto others as you would have them do unto you" is, of course, what this means. For instance, respect for other people leads to respect for oneself.

Niyama
Niyama is the name of the second limb. Self-control and spiritual observances are the focal points of this limb. For instance, it is crucial to observe spiritual health and well-being to attend a house of worship and say grace before eating. Similar to this, going on regular walks by yourself or engaging in meditation help you connect with the essence of your own being and discover your purpose for being on Earth.

In Asana
Asanas is the name of the third limb. These are the yoga poses that are practiced, with the belief that the body is the temple of the spirit. From a yogic perspective, asanas enhance our general health, discipline, attention, and spiritual development. The ability to meditate and focus inward for harmony, tranquility, and happiness on the inside as well as the outside is another crucial function of asanas.

Pranayama
Pranayama is the name of the fourth limb. This is basically breath control, which is meant to regulate and master our breathing abilities. We also discover the link between breathing and life, as well as how healthy breathing may elevate our mental and emotional states. Pranayama, which means "life force extension," is a yoga pose that some think nourishes and revitalizes the body,

mind, and soul or spirit. You can incorporate this method into your regular yoga practice or use it on its own.

Prityahara

Pratyahara is the fifth limb of yoga. This basically refers to retreating from the outside world, surroundings, and stimulus. Pratyahara is a deliberate attempt to achieve a state of detachment from our senses as a type of sensory transcendence. We focus entirely inward when we use this strategy. This helps us to take a step back from daily life and examine ourselves within. Additionally, we gain insight into our behaviors and urges, which may be detrimental to our general health, wellbeing, and well-being.

Dharane

Yoga's sixth limb is called dharana. It's critical to understand that every yoga limb or level advances us to the next. In light of this, dharana, or concentration, comes after pratyahara. With the help of this limb, we can overcome the outside influences, digressions, and other distractions that cloud our regular thinking. Additionally, it establishes the foundation for appropriate meditation methods. Dharana helps us strengthen our ability to focus while teaching us how to slow down the thought process. With this, we may take charge of our thoughts and brains instead of letting them rule us. You will effortlessly enter a daily state of extended meditation after you have mastered this technique.

Dharamendra

The seventh limb of yoga, dhyana, is centered on the unbroken flow of focus. Dharana is referred to as concentration, and dhyana as meditation. Though there is a thin line separating these limbs, these stages are also interwoven. As an illustration, dharana is the practice of achieving one-pointed attention, whereas dhyana is the awareness without focus. Your mind is calm and you have few or no thoughts when you are in a dhyana state.

At this point, you also have increased strength and endurance. But yoga itself is about discipline, daily instruction, and following—not perfection.

This suggests that nothing is ever impossible to accomplish, but if you are unable to do something, it's acceptable to go on with your life. Whatever your level of experience or expertise, yoga offers mental and physical health advantages at every step.

In Samadhi

Samadhi is the eighth and final limb or stage of yoga. This is a naturally occurring ecstatic condition in which the practitioner feels a connection to the Divine. In this level of meditation, which is also regarded as the final one, your attention and point of view have become one with the self. Recall that yoga is something that can only be experienced, not "mastered" per se. This holds true for every stage that leads up to spiritual awareness.

Yoga Types

Selecting a yoga style that aligns with your abilities and objectives will yield the best results among the various forms of yoga. For those who are new to yoga, hatha yoga is an excellent beginning. Try this relaxed method of breathing and stretching if you're just starting out or have never done yoga before. It will feel soothing and rejuvenating to you.

Another well-liked style of yoga is Vinyasa. This works very well for because of your regular movement, those who are attempting to lose weight from one stance and one pose to the next. Thus, you receive a little amount of a combine an aerobic workout with your yoga routine. Burning up to seven calories per minute by alternating between lunges, floor exercises, and stances when standing.

Additionally, Bikram yoga will increase your flexibility and help you lose weight. That's utilized in "hot yoga" workouts, in which participants work out in rooms that are It was scorching. It is considered beneficial by practitioners to sweat off the body's poisons and pollutants when practicing yoga.

Advantages of Yoga

Your physical, mental, and emotional well-being will benefit greatly from yoga practice. You can utilize it to feel lighter, stronger, and more youthful.

It gives you a comprehensive approach to physical fitness and well-being in addition to stretching your body, burning calories, and improving your appearance. Your body becomes open, flexible, and in harmony with your mind and heart via yoga. It's a terrific way to add some extra fitness to an already established routine and is especially beneficial for those who want to concentrate on breathing, stretching, and reaching that elusive inner calm.

Benefits of Yoga for Losing Weight: Body

Few individuals are aware of yoga's potential as an effective calorie burner. You won't be hopping around and perspiring as you would when playing basketball, running, or cross training. Every time you practice yoga for thirty or sixty minutes, you do, in fact, burn calories consistently. You can burn about 300 calories in an hour with even a basic yoga practice that incorporates poses and stances from Hatha yoga. You will be able to burn even more if you decide to step it up and practice a more vigorous style of yoga, like Vinyasa or Ashtanga. There is always a chance to burn calories when moving.

Yoga also plays a crucial role in helping you lose weight by raising your body awareness. You must pay attention to your body's movements and actions in every pose and position. You'll be aware of the way your body functions as a whole and have a deep awareness of every muscle and limb.

Practicing yoga greatly enhances flexibility. Your ability to move and maintain balance will improve as a result of all of your stretching. It will become easier for you to breathe and move, and your posture will also get better. Although it may not seem like it would be crucial for weight loss, this does. Your degree of physical fitness automatically rises when you can move with greater ease. This keeps you active and helps you lose body fat. Being more flexible leads to improved fitness. You'll discover that even accomplishing basic tasks makes you feel better and that you look better in your clothes.

Benefits of Yoga for Losing Weight: Mind

Yoga combines mental, emotional, and physical well-being. Positive thinking plays a major role in weight loss success. You are teaching your mind to harness the power of intention and positivity when you include a daily yoga practice into your weight reduction regimen. You can use the time you spend stretching and holding poses to imagine yourself as healthier, stronger, and thinner. You'll experience weight loss more naturally if you live in an expectant state. Yoga will assist you in connecting with and utilizing your intention, as the mind is a potent tool in the fight against weight loss.

In addition to eliminating bad food and upping physical exercise, controlling stress is a key component of weight management. An emotional imbalance can lead to poor habits when you feel overwhelmed or frightened. Yoga helps you stay at ease and teaches you how to guide yourself back to serenity when stress begins to overwhelm your body and mind. You'll stay optimistic and in balance if you practice mindfulness.

Practicing yoga is a life-changing, uplifting practice. You'll see immediate improvements in your appearance and well-being, regardless of whether you're starting out or enhancing an existing practice.

7

Yoga Training Program for Novices

Week One

Yoga is a practice that may be done practically anywhere, without the need for any equipment, and without any prerequisite knowledge. For these reasons, this is a great workout to start with and perfect for those who want to practice at home. Yoga trousers, leggings, or shorts are helpful, as is a top that is cozy but not too big, however there aren't really any rules when it comes to attire. Not only should you practice on a mat or towel, but you should also practice barefoot.

During the course of these two weeks, you will learn and practice new, basic yoga poses every day. On Sundays, you will review all of the poses you have learned thus far. The starting and finishing poses for every yoga session will be taught to you on the first day.

Monday, Week 1: Corpse and Easy Pose

The Easy stance is the first stance you should master. You will start each session in this posture.

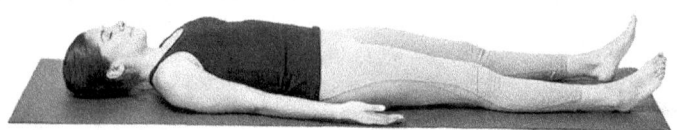

1. Take a seat and start with your legs extended in front of you, crossed at the shins.

2. With your legs folded in toward you and your knees wide, place each foot under the knee of the person on the opposite side.

3. With your palms facing up or down, place your hands on your knees.

4. Sit up straight and equally distribute your weight across your hip bones.

5. Stretch out your back and erect your head, neck, and spine.

6. Extend your chest forth and lower your shoulders back.

7. Inhale deeply and maintain this position for fifteen minutes.

The Corpse Pose is the second posture to master. Every class will conclude with this pose, which is regarded as the most crucial to learn.

YOGA TRAINING PROGRAM FOR NOVICES

Corpse Pose
Savasana

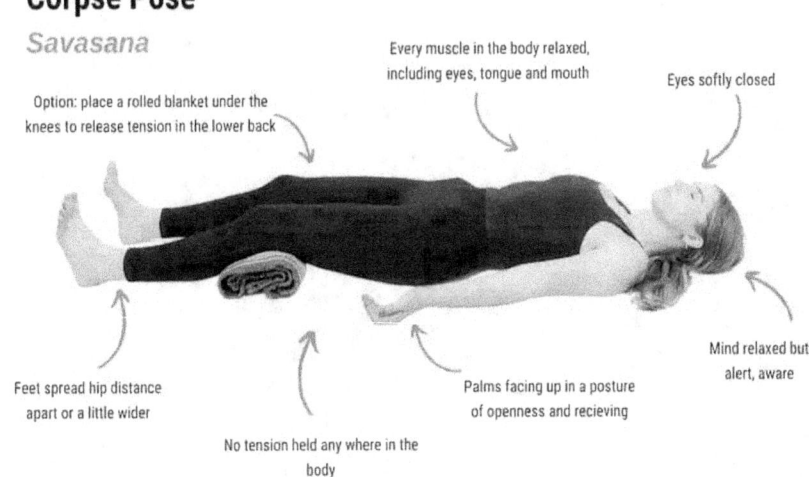

1. Lay flat on your back with your arms six inches from your sides and your palms facing up.

2. Inhale organically.

3. After closing your eyes, deliberately start to relax every muscle in your body, starting from your head and ending at the base of your feet.

4. Maintain this position for fifteen minutes at a time.

Tuesday: Handstand in the mountain

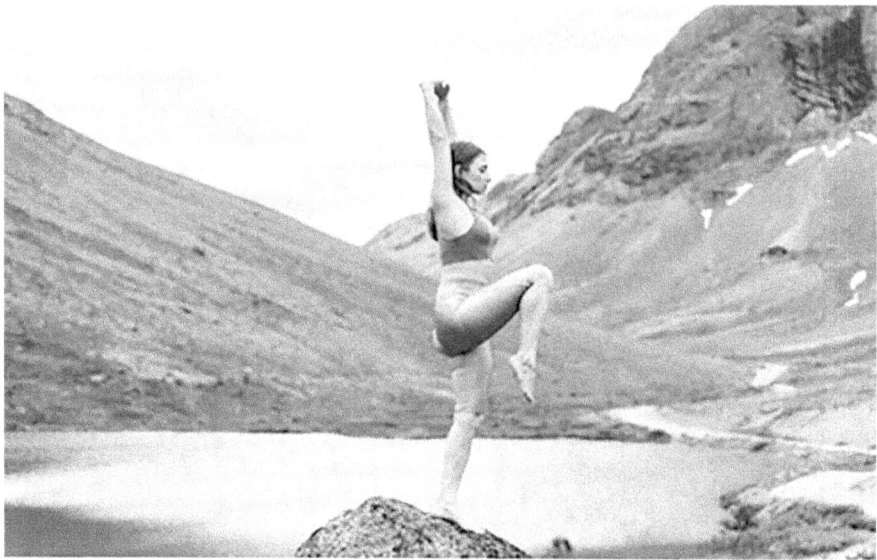

1. Take five minutes to hold the Easy Pose at the beginning.
2. Take a tall stance and place your feet hip-width apart to begin the Mountain Pose.
3. Maintain a balanced weight distribution, relaxed shoulders, and arms at your sides.
4. Exhale deeply and lift your hands, extending your fingers upwards.
5. Breathe gently while holding for up to a minute.
6. Return to the initial position and perform the stretch many times with your hands by your sides.
7. Complete five minutes in corpse pose.

Wednesday: Cobra stance

1. Take five minutes to hold the Easy Pose at the beginning.
2. Step into Warrior Pose by placing your feet three to four feet apart.
3. Bring your left foot in slightly with your right foot turned 90 degrees.
4. Extend yourself to your sides, hands down, while maintaining a relaxed posture and lowered shoulders at the hips.
5. Maintaining your knee over your ankle, bend your right knee to a 90-

degree angle.

6. Take a minute to gaze over your right hand and maintain the stance.
7. Change sides and continue for however many times you like.

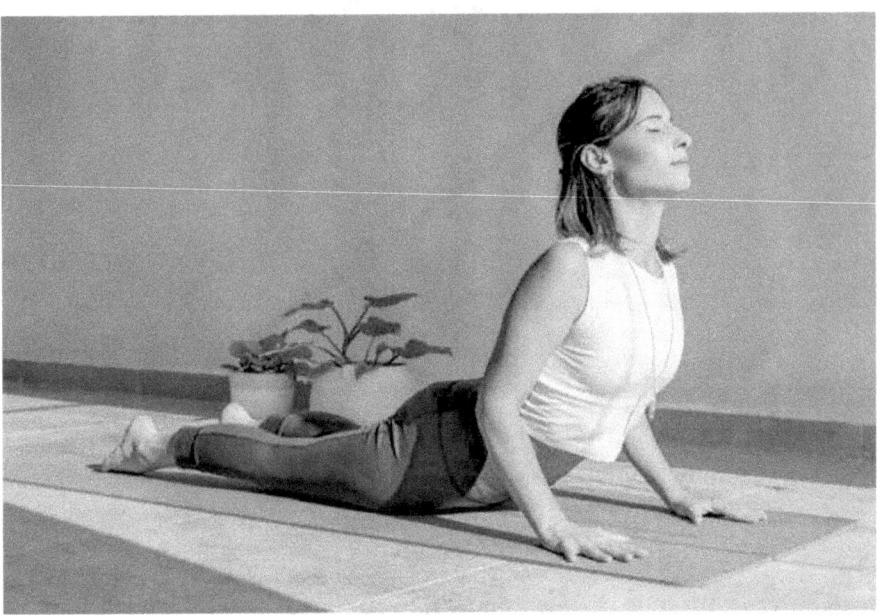

8. Close with five minutes in corpse pose.

Downward Dog on Thursday

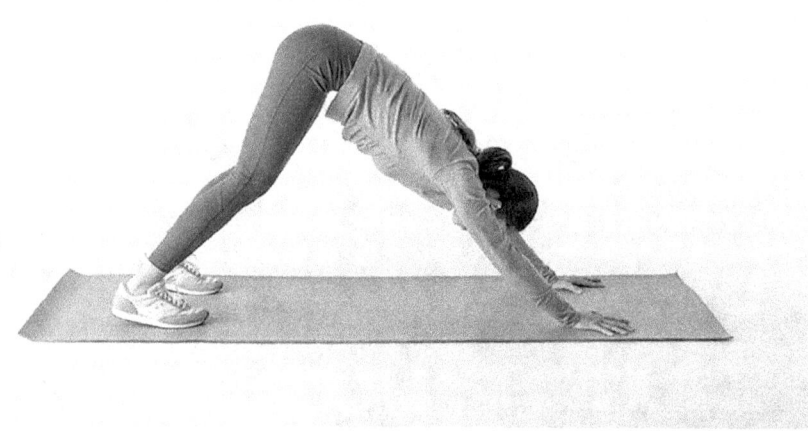

1. Take five minutes to hold the Easy Pose at the beginning.

2. On the floor, begin Downward Dog by getting on your hands and knees.

3. Place your hands beneath your shoulders and your knees beneath your hips.

4. Spread your fingers widely and walk your hands slowly forward, keeping your palms level on the ground.

5. Your body should resemble an inverted V as you raise your hips and curl your toes under while slightly bending your knees.

6. Take three deep breaths and maintain this stance. You have as many opportunities as you wish to repeat the entire process.

7. Complete five minutes in corpse pose.

Tree Pose on Friday

1. Take five minutes to hold the Easy Pose at the beginning.

2. With your arms by your sides, adopt the Tree Pose by standing tall and straight.

3. Maintaining your forward posture, transfer your weight to your left leg

and position your foot's bottom within your left thigh.

4. Maintain your balance and raise your hands in front of you in the stance of prayer, palms facing each other.

5. Take a deep breath, raise your arms over your shoulders, keep your palms facing apart, and hold the position for thirty seconds.

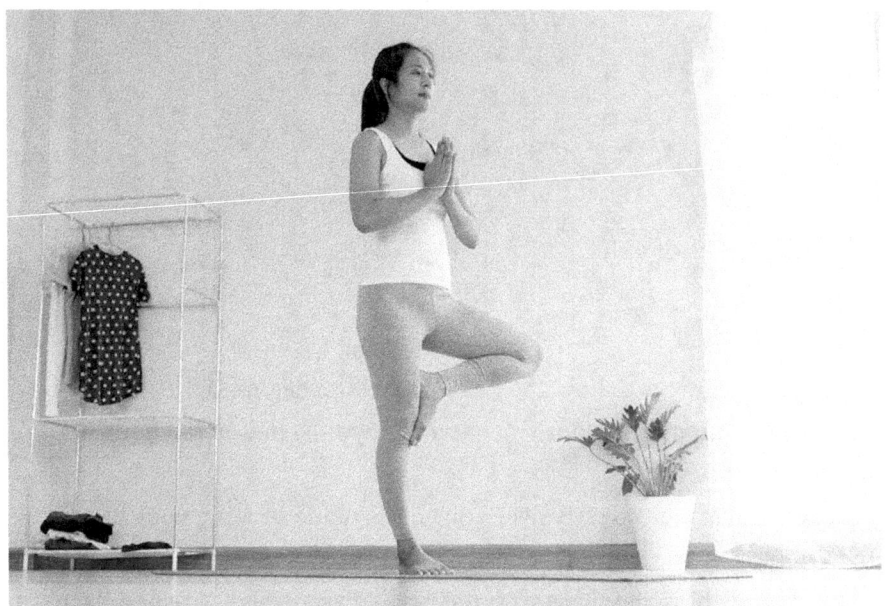

6. Lower your arms, then repeat on the other side.

7. Continue for as long as you like, switching between the left and right sides.

8. Close with five minutes in corpse pose.

Bridge Pose on Saturday.

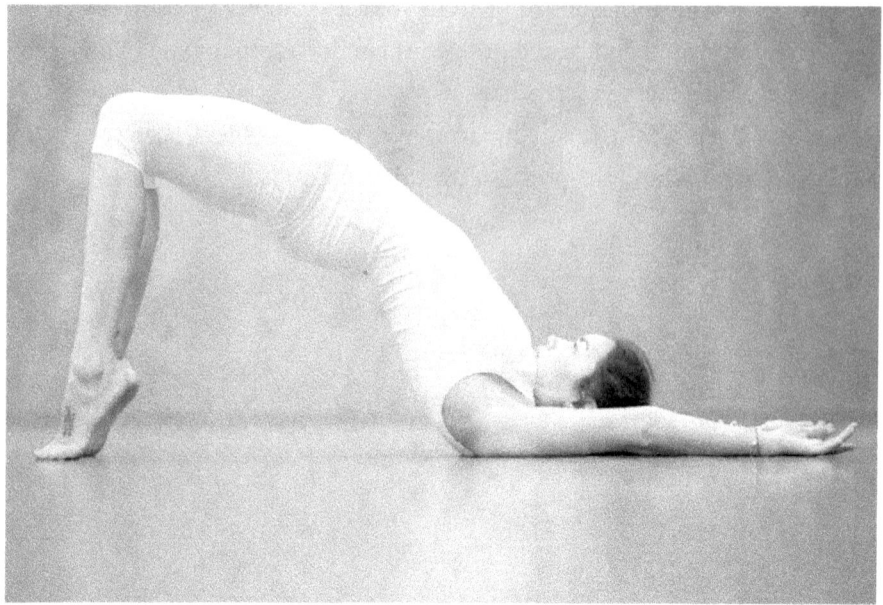

1. Take five minutes to hold the Easy Pose at the beginning.

2. Place your arms at your sides and your palms flat on the floor to begin the Bridge Pose.

3. Set your knees directly over your heels while keeping your feet flat on the ground.

4. Lift your hips and plant your feet so that your thighs are parallel to the floor as you release the breath.

5. Fold your hands beneath your lower back and tuck your arms under.

6. Remain in the stance for one minute, then switch it up as many as you wish.

7. Complete five minutes in corpse pose.

Sunday: Child's Pose and the First Week Review

Begin in Easy Pose and hold it for one minute. Then, progress to Warrior Pose, Downward Dog, Mountain Pose, Tree Pose, and Bridge Pose. Make sure to perform Warrior and Tree poses for one minute on both the right and left sides. Proceed to Sunday's new stance, Child stance, after the review, and conclude as usual with Corpse Pose.

Infant Pose

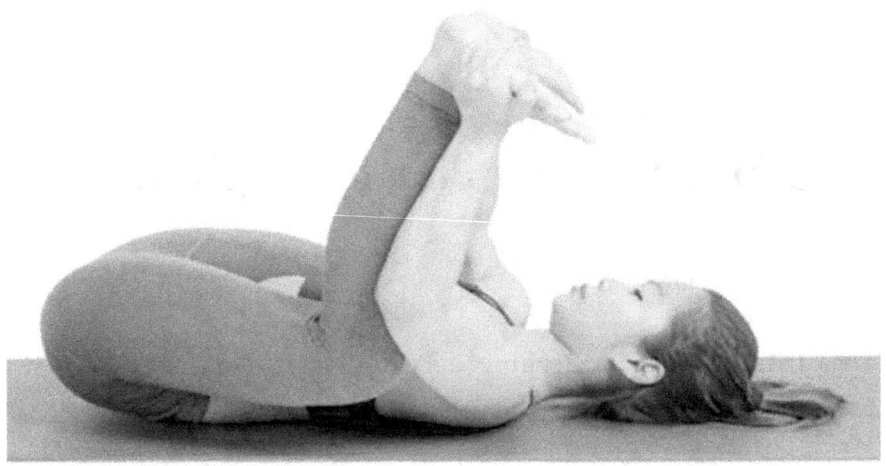

1. Start Child's Pose by sitting up straight on your heels following the Week 1 Review.

2. Extend your body forward such that your forehead rests on the ground in front of you.

3. As close to comfortably as possible, lower your chest to your knees, then raise your arms straight up in front of you.

4. Lay your palms down flat on the floor.

Take a deep breath and maintain this stance for a minute. You can practice this pose as many times as you wish.

6. Take a minute to end in corpse pose.

8

Yoga Training Plan for Beginners

Yoga Training Plan for Beginners: Two Weeks:

Week Two

Every day in the second week, you will learn a new stance, and at the conclusion of the week, you will review every pose you learned in the second week.

Monday: Pose in Triangles

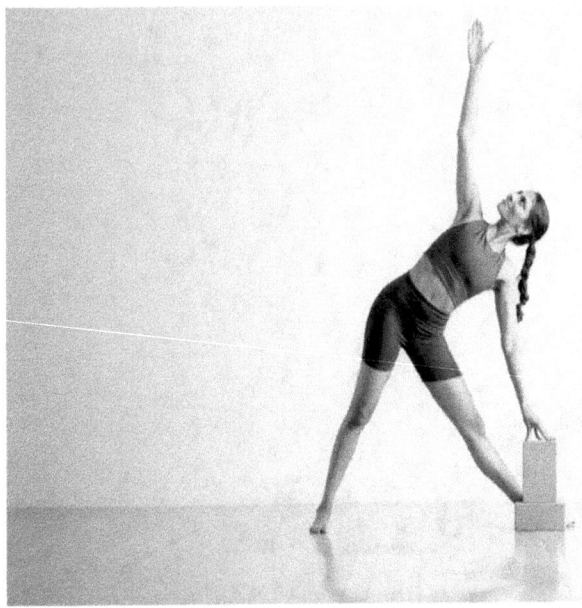

1. Take five minutes to hold the Easy Pose at the beginning.
2. To begin Triangle Pose, stand upright with your arms out to your sides and your feet shoulder-width apart.
3. Extend your left foot 45 degrees and your right foot 90 degrees.
4. With your legs straight, touch your right hand to your right foot.
5. Look up past your left hand as you reach for the sky, and hold there for five breaths.
6. Carry out step 6 on the other side.
7. Continue for as long as you like, switching between the left and right sides.
8. Close with five minutes in corpse pose.

Tuesday: Dog with an upward face

WOMEN'S EXERCISE PROGRAMS

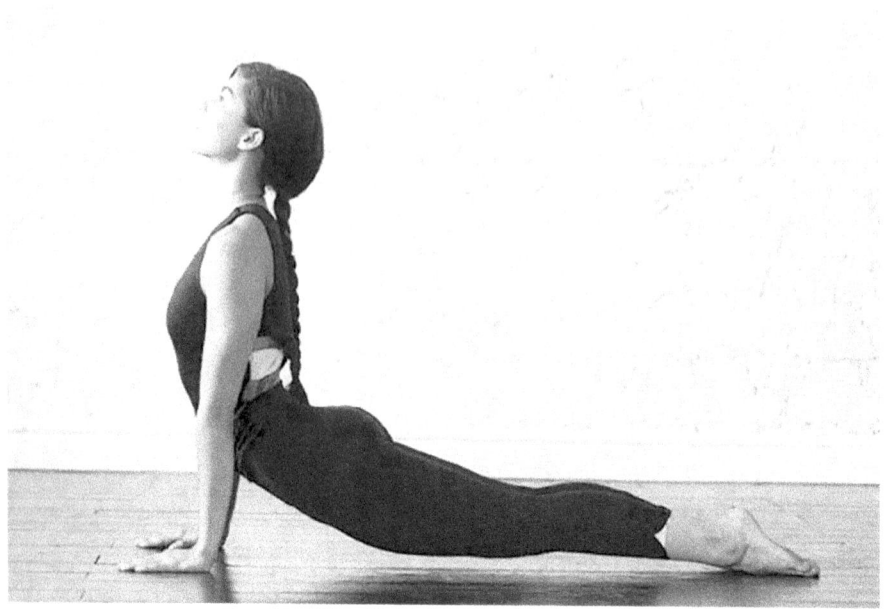

1. Take five minutes to hold the Easy Pose at the beginning.

2. Begin by lying face down on the floor in the Upward Facing Dog pose.

3. Immediately beneath your shoulders, place your hands, palms down, flat on the ground.

4. With the tops of your feet still on the ground, extend your legs behind you.

5. Squeeze your rear end and tighten your pelvic floor by tucking your hips down.

6. Maintain your hips on the ground while pressing your hands into the earth and lifting your chest off the ground.

7. Keep your grip for a minute, then release it and repeat as many as desired.

8. Close with five minutes in corpse pose.

Wednesday: Twist in a chair

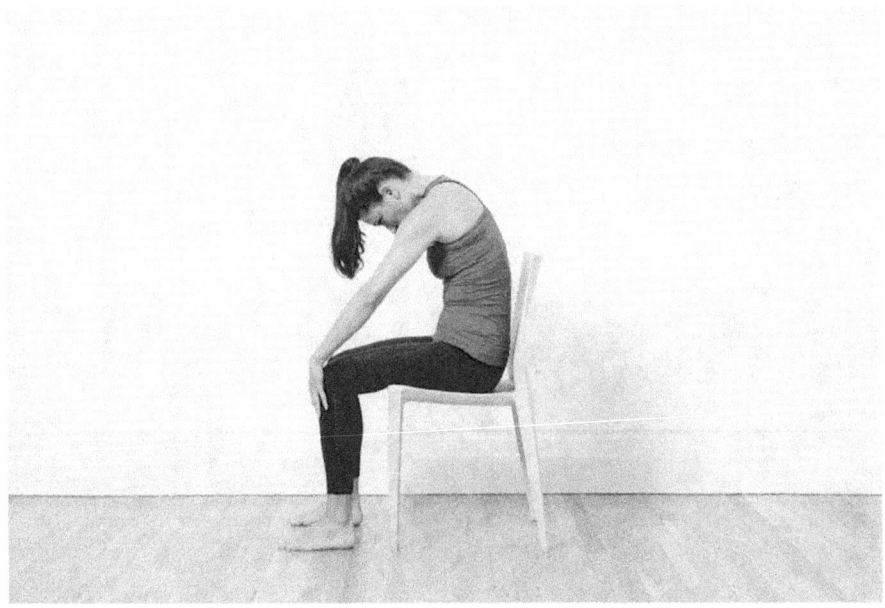

1. Take five minutes to hold the Easy Pose at the beginning.
2. Sit on the floor with your legs out straight in front of you to begin the Seated Twist.
3. Place your right foot outside the length of your left thigh.
4. Bend your left knee and raise your right knee to the sky.
5. Place your left elbow outside of your right knee while supporting yourself with your right hand on the floor.
6. Maintain your glutes on the ground and, starting from your abdomen, twist to the right as far as feels comfortable.
7. Hold for one minute or longer.
8. Transition to the other side.
9. Continue for as long as you like, switching between the left and right sides.
10. Spend five minutes in corpse pose to finish.

Pigeon pose on Thursday

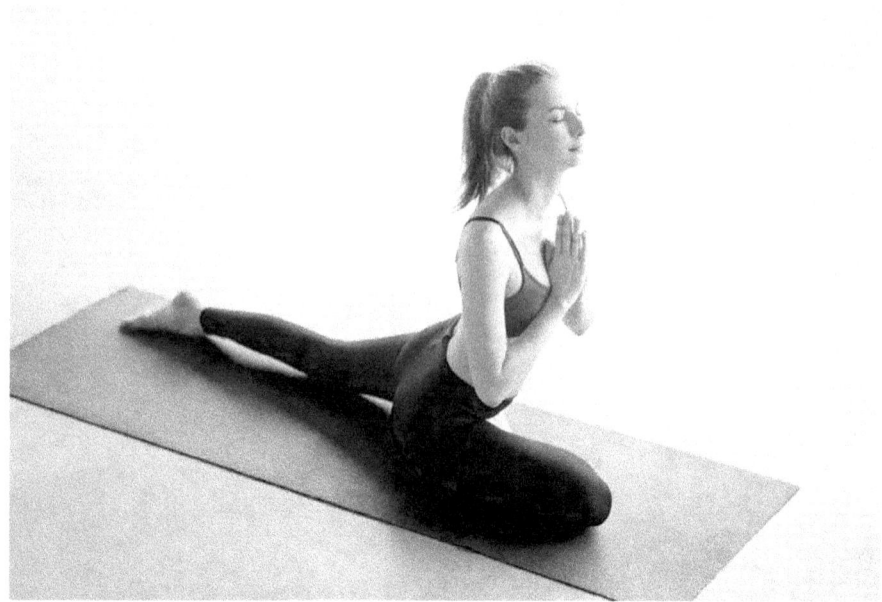

1. Take five minutes to hold the Easy Pose at the beginning.

2. Place your hands directly beneath your shoulders, palms down, to begin Pigeon Pose from a push-up position.

3. Bring your left knee up to your shoulder on the floor. Your right hip should be next to your left heel.

4. Lift your chest by pressing your hands into the ground, then recline.

5. Maintain the posture for a maximum of one minute.

6. Make the switch to the other side.

7. Continue for as long as you like, switching between the left and right sides.

8. Close with five minutes in corpse pose.

Friday: Pose like a dolphin

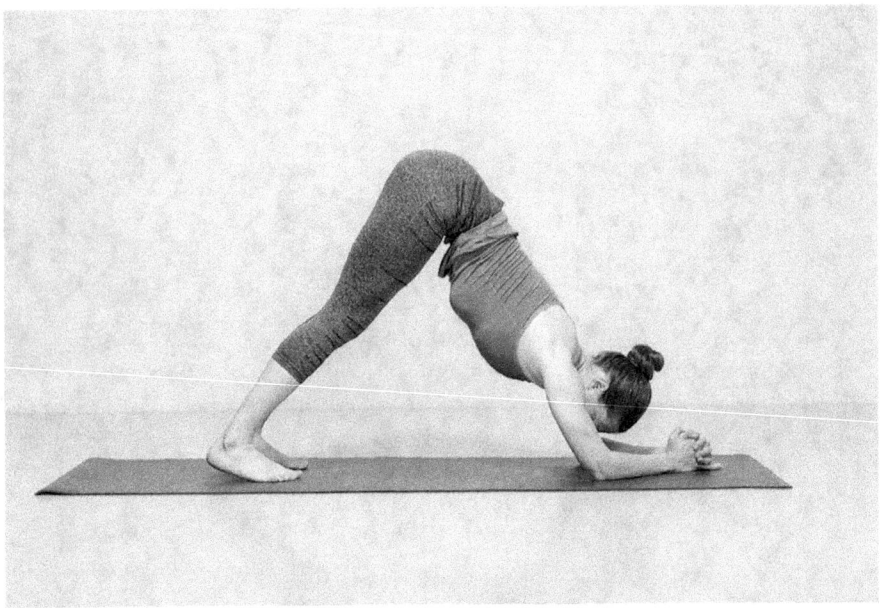

1. Take five minutes to hold the Easy Pose at the beginning.

2. Come into Downward Dog Pose to begin Dolphin Pose.

3. Lie on your back with your forearms pointing down.

4. Maintaining your hands shoulder-width apart, spread your fingers widely.

5. Breathe deeply, plant your forehead on the ground, and hold the position for a minute.

6. Complete five minutes in corpse pose.

Half Wheel Pose on Saturday.

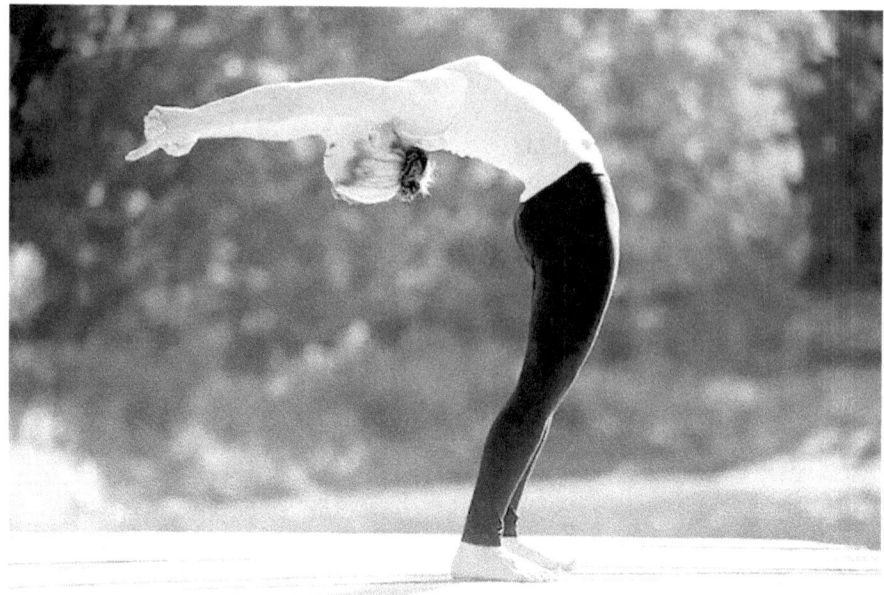

1. Take five minutes to hold the Easy Pose at the beginning.

2. Start in Bridge Pose, then transition into Half Wheel Pose.

3. Ascend as high as you can on your toes alone after shifting off the heels of your feet in the bridge position.

4. Maintain a flat palm position and keep your arms on the ground. Take a minute or so to maintain this posture.

5. Complete five minutes in corpse pose.

Sunday: Review of Week Two and Boat Pose

Easy Pose should be held for one minute at a time. After that, hold Triangle Pose, Upward Facing Dog, Seated Twist, Pigeon Pose, Dolphin Pose, and Half Wheel Pose for a minute each. Make sure to complete the Triangle, Seated Twist, and Pigeon poses for one minute on both the right and left sides. Proceed to Sunday's new pose, Boat Pose, after the review, and finish as usual with Corpse Pose.

Floating Position

YOGA TRAINING PLAN FOR BEGINNERS

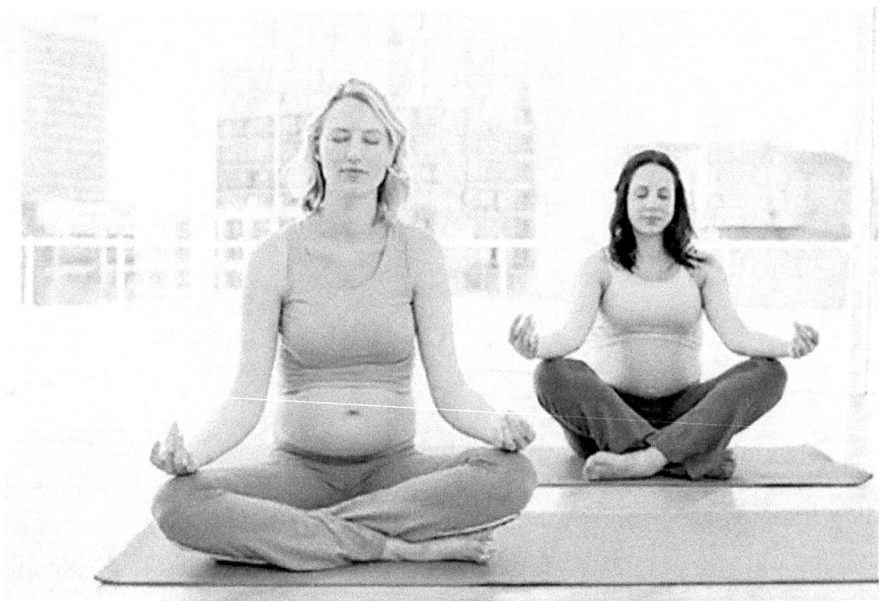

1. To begin Boat Pose, after Week 2 Review, sit on the floor with your legs out in front of you.

2. Maintain a straight posture and squeeze your legs together.

3. Form a V with your body by lifting your knees off the ground and leaning slightly back while maintaining your arms parallel to your body for balance.

4. Maintain the stance for as long as you can while noticing how your thighs and tummy muscles are keeping you still.

5. Let go and repeat the pose as many times as desired.

6. Take a minute to end in corpse pose.

Following the second week, you can repeat this training program at two-week intervals or design your own using the positions you find most comfortable.

9

Advice for Novices in Yoga

Beginning yoga is exhilarating. If this is something you have never done before and you are unsure of what to anticipate, you should be willing to work at your own pace and maintain an open mind. You don't have to become proficient in the trickiest postures and poses straight away. You will discover several pointers in this chapter that will equip you with the resources and self-assurance you want to get going. Stick with it is the most crucial piece of advice. Making the commitment to practice yoga for weight loss and overall wellness is a wise decision that will pay off in the long run. Yoga isn't a trendy workout or a passing craze. You'll quickly discover that it's a way of life.

Ways to Proceed

Finding a friend is among the most crucial things you can accomplish. When practiced alone, yoga is a very effective practice; however, when you have a partner, it becomes an enjoyable social activity that also serves health benefits. If no one is willing to practice yoga with you, sign up for a session that happens once a week at the very least. Many others who share your interests will approach you and be eager to assist you in developing your yoga practice.

Another important "to do" is to set aside space in your house for yoga. You don't need a yoga studio set up with mirrors on every wall and a stack of mats for this. Even when you're attending courses at a gym or studio, having a small space where you can stretch when you're agitated will be beneficial. Pay attention to both the physical and mental aspects of yoga.

Both in and out of the classroom, you'll be moving and stretching a lot. Make the time to meditate, focus on your breathing, engage in positive thinking, and visualize a happy life. Every day, your yoga practice should be a part of your life.

What Not to Do

Avoid comparing yourself to other people. It might be difficult to maintain even the most basic version of Mountain Pose if you're new to yoga. That's alright. That one posture can take up a whole day, or perhaps a week, to practice. You're not up against anyone, and there's no time limit. Those who are further along in life should inspire and motivate you; however, resist the need to give in to feelings of inferiority or insecurity.

Be careful not to overreact. Burnout is a common outcome of trying to do too much too soon. As your body becomes used to the additional demands you're placing on it, gradually increase the length of your workouts from 30 to 60 minutes three times a week.

Reject any negativity that can hinder you. Thank your well-meaning friends for their advice when they try to convince you that practicing yoga won't help you lose weight, and then keep going. You may improve your health and waistline without having to spend hours lifting weights or running marathons.

Required Financial Outlays

Start assembling a library. Invest in films and DVDs, read books and publications. Get some CDs and read blogs on yoga. In addition to keeping you informed and educated, these items will inspire you.

Invest on a quality matting. An uncomfortable class versus a fun one can be determined by your yoga mat. Try a couple yoga mats before you buy; there are plenty of them available on the market. Ask others about the mats they use to learn what and why they appreciate it. Buy yoga clothing that fits properly, wicks away moisture, and lets you breathe.

For your body to flow effortlessly through your poses, you should wear fitted tops, shorts, and pants. But anything that is too tight will feel uncomfortable.

Consciously Eating

When starting yoga, it's crucial to get plenty of rest. Both your physical and mental well-being require recuperation. Eating a healthy diet plays a significant role in maintaining your body's strength and alignment with the positive energy flow you are attempting to create. You already know the basic rules of weight loss: consume foods that make you feel good about yourself rather than depressing you and burn more calories than you consume. You should establish for yourself a few basic eating guidelines. These instructions will not only help you reduce your weight but also improve your physical preparedness for yoga.

With Awareness When Eating

When you first start practicing yoga, it's crucial to obtain plenty of sleep. Both physical and mental recuperation are necessary. Maintaining the strength and alignment of your body with the positive energy flow you are attempting to create is also greatly influenced by the food you eat. You already know the fundamentals of weight loss: consume foods that increase rather than decrease your body's capacity to burn calories. It is necessary for you to establish a few basic eating guidelines. These tips won't just aid in weight loss; they'll also improve your body's suitability for yoga.

Remove the clutter. Simply refuse processed foods that are high in sugar, sodium, and fat, as well as fast food and packaged goods. Stay away from them. You are learning the skill of balancing your mind, body, and spirit when you practice yoga. Fast meals will make you slower.

Rather, concentrate on what's in season, local, and fresh. When you're hungry, stuff yourself with fruits and veggies. That need to be your first goal, whether it's a springtime bunch of luscious berries or a fall clementine orange. Start going to your neighborhood farmer's market on a regular basis.

You can do yoga with more energy if you eat lean protein. Add skinless chicken breasts, eggs, almonds, and healthy fat-rich oils to your cooking, along with omega-rich fish like sardines and salmon. If you're a vegetarian, you'll need to obtain your protein from other foods, such as tofu, beans and legumes, and robust veggies like squash, eggplant, and mushrooms.

In conclusion

This book will help you get the most out of the beginning of your yoga practice. Stay enthusiastic and full of energy as you become enthused about all the fascinating things yoga can teach you about your body and health. This workout is distinct from other types. It reaches into your soul and changes your perspective on everything, even dieting and losing weight. Be willing to go wherever this adventure leads you, and keep your body and mind open. Lastly, let me express my gratitude for having read my book. Please take a moment to write a review and share your opinions about the book on Amazon if you liked it. I would be really grateful for that!